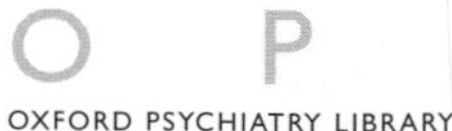

OXFORD PSYCHIATRY LIBRARY

Depression in Later Life

O P L

OXFORD PSYCHIATRY LIBRARY

Depression in Later Life

Second Edition

Robert C. Baldwin

Consultant Old Age Psychiatrist and
Honorary Professor of Psychiatry,
Manchester Mental Health and Social Care Trust,
Park House
North Manchester General Hospital,
Manchester, UK

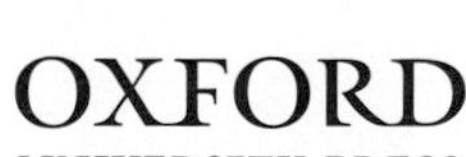

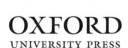

OXFORD
UNIVERSITY PRESS

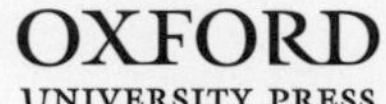

Great Clarendon Street, Oxford, OX2 6DP,
United Kingdom

Oxford University Press is a department of the University of Oxford. It furthers the University's objective of excellence in research, scholarship, and education by publishing worldwide. Oxford is a registered trade mark of Oxford University Press in the UK and in certain other countries

Impression: 1

Published in the United States of America by Oxford University Press
198 Madison Avenue, New York, NY 10016, United States of America

British Library Cataloguing in Publication Data
Data available

Library of Congress Control Number: 2013955309

ISBN 978–0–19–967163–2

Printed in Great Britain by
Ashford Colour Press Ltd, Gosport, Hampshire

Contents

Symbols and Abbreviations

α	alpha
≥	equal to/greater than
>	greater than
<	less than
%	per cent
ACE	angiotensin-converting enzyme
ADH	antidiuretic hormone
AIDS	acquired immunodeficiency syndrome
BABCP	British Association of Behavioural and Cognitive Psychotherapies
BAP	British Association of Psychopharmacology
bd	*bis in die* (twice daily)
CANMAT	Canadian Network for Mood and Anxiety Treatments
CBT	cognitive behavioural therapy
CG	clinical guideline
CHD	coronary heart disease
CNS	central nervous system
COPD	chronic obstructive pulmonary disease
CRF	corticotropin-releasing factor
CT	computerized tomography
DALY	disability adjusted life year
DEDS	depression-executive dysfunction syndrome
DSM	Diagnostic and Statistical Manual
ECG	electrocardiogram
ECT	electroconvulsive treatment
EEG	electroencephalogram
FSC	fronto-striatal circuit
GDS	geriatric depression scale
GHRF	growth hormone-releasing factor
GI	gastrointestinal
GP	general practitioner
HADS	hospital anxiety and depression scale
HDRS	Hamilton depression rating scale
HIV	human immunodeficiency virus
HPA	hypothalamic-pituitary-adrenal

5HT	5-hydroxytryptamine
IADH	inappropriate antidiuretic hormone
IAPT	Improving Access to Psychological Therapies
ICD	International Classification of Diseases
IPT	interpersonal therapy
kg	kilogram
L	litre
lb	pound
MADRAS	Montgomery-Äsberg depression rating scale
MAO-A	monoamine oxidase A
MAOI	monoamine oxidase inhibitor
MCI	mild cognitive impairment
mg	milligram
MHRA	Medicines and Health products Regulatory Authority
mmol	millimole
MoCA	Montreal cognitive assessment
MRI	magnetic resonance imaging
mRNA	messenger ribonucleic acid
ms	millisecond
NARI	noradrenaline reuptake inihibitor
NASSa	noradrenaline and specific serotonin antidepressant
NICE	National Institute for Health and Care Excellence
NSAID	non-steroidal anti-inflammatory drug
OMC	orientation-memory-concentration
PET	positron emission tomography
PHQ	patient health questionnaire
PST	problem-solving treatment
rCBF	regional cerebral blood flow
RCT	randomized controlled trial
rTMS	repetitive transcranial magnetic stimulation
SNRI	serotonin/noradrenaline reuptake inhibitor
SPECT	single photon emission computerized tomography
SSRI	selective serotonin reuptake inhibitor
TCA	tricyclic antidepressant
tds	*ter die sumendum* (three times daily)
TRH	thyrotropin-releasing hormone
UK	United Kingdom
US	United States
WML	white matter lesion

Chapter 1

Introduction

Lilly is 88, and her daily requests to be taken to see a doctor about her 'stomach wind' are wearing out her 60-year-old recently retired son, who is finding himself waking early in the morning with worry. John is 72 and devastated at the unexpected loss of his wife just before their 50th wedding anniversary. His family and friends are sympathetic, but, 6 months on, he is fretful, miserable and feels he will burden people by talking about it. Wong-Chai has had arthritis for the last 20 of her 75 years. Once proud and indomitable, she has lately found her joint pain unbearable and has wondered about 'going to sleep and never waking up'. Raj is 85 and lately finds himself unable to concentrate, so much so that he keeps losing things. His sleep and appetite are poor, and he has stopped going to the local day care centre. His doctor said it is his age, but his family fear the start of dementia. Jack, aged 76, has turned up in the emergency department, feeling nauseous and dizzy. Recently, he has lost weight and feels very tired, lonely, and miserable. He admits to taking four sleeping tablets last night 'just to get a bit of peace for the night'. The doctor tells him not to worry—that dose will not harm him. A week later, he is back with a serious paracetamol overdose.

What links these vignettes is depressive disorder. Although dementia is regarded as the typical mental health condition of later life, in fact, depression is more common. Often overlooked, depression is a very serious problem in later life. It reduces the quality of life and adds to the disability associated with all the major medical illnesses that afflict older people. It often complicates the course of dementia as well as being a risk factor for it.

Epitomized by the statement 'Who would not be depressed at that age?', it is tempting, but completely inaccurate, to assume that depression must be the norm in later life. In the main, health professionals see older people who are most susceptible to depression, those with frailty and chronic medical illnesses. The trap is to 'normalize' depression in ill older people, with the result that major depression can be overlooked. In reality, many older people live contentedly, with their quality of life improving with age (Netuveli *et al.* 2006). Of those who do become depressed, many have a diagnosable mental health disorder, and there are interventions which can help significantly.

There are already textbooks on depression; why then is one needed specifically for depression in later life? First, there is the self-evident fact that the world's population is fast growing older. This brings with it increasing rates of many of the common health problems, including depression. Second, although depression in later life shares many of the core features with depression at other times, there are some important differences. Third, late-life depression frequently occurs in the setting of significant medical morbidity which complicates both the diagnosis and treatment. Last, depression in this age group often presents with altered cognition, and unravelling mood from memory impairment requires skill.

This book sets out the core knowledge about late-life depressive disorders and summarizes the key evidence base for successful interventions relevant to practitioners who work with older people.

Key references

Netuveli G, Wiggins RD, Hildon Z, Montgomery SM, Blane D (2006). Quality of life at older ages: evidence from the English longitudinal study of aging (wave 1). *Journal of Epidemiology and Community Health*, **60**, 357–63.

Chapter 2

Classification and epidemiology

Key points

- Current classificatory systems for depression underestimate the level of depression among older people.
- In later life, the impact of having even just a few persistent symptoms of depression is considerable.
- Poor health is strongly linked to depressive disorder in later life so that care homes and acute hospitals have an especially high prevalence.
- Depressive disorder adds to the morbidity of many common medical disorders of later life.
- In later life, be especially vigilant for organic causes of depression (systemic illness, cerebral disease, medication, alcohol).

2.1 Types of depression in later life

Depression can mean a symptom or a syndrome. As a **symptom**, the key to distinguishing morbid depression from the transitory low mood experienced by everyone from time to time is that, in depression, there is a qualitative change in mood. Those affected recognize this change in mood themselves. They may also be aware that the duration and frequency differ (most days, most of the time) from transient unhappiness and that even positive events produce little relief.

In recent years, there has been a significant change in how depression is conceptualized. Rather than fixed categories of depression into which the patient must be squeezed, the evidence suggests that depression is on a continuum, from normal sadness to pathologically severe depression (Paykel and Priest 1992). Nevertheless, in psychiatry, as in the rest of medicine, practice would be impossible without some kind of classification, and the most common approach is to set a threshold of symptoms above which a patient is said to have the **syndrome** of depression (see Box 2.1). The threshold is set by criteria agreed via one of the two international systems of classification, the International Classification of Diseases (ICD-10) (World Health Organization 1994) or the Diagnostic and Statistical Manual (DSM-V) (American Psychiatric Association 2013). Although broadly similar, the latter is easier to grasp and, according to evidence from treatment trials, more efficient in treatment decisions. The previous DSM classification (DSM-IV) is used by the English National Institute for Health and Care Excellence. The DSM-V scheme is outlined in Box 2.1 and specifies that five core symptoms must be present and one must be depressed mood or loss of interest or pleasure. These

Box 2.1 DSM-V criteria for major depressive disorder (American Psychiatric Association 2013)

Three domains A–C must be covered before a diagnosis of major depression can be made.

A. Five or more of the core symptoms present during the same 2-week period, with a change from previous functioning; at least one of the symptoms must be either (1) depressed mood or (2) loss of interest or pleasure. The core symptoms are:

(1) Depressed mood most of the day, nearly every day, as indicated by either subjective report or noted by others (for example, tearfulness).

(2) Markedly diminished interest or pleasure involving all, or almost all, activities most of the time.

(3) Significant weight loss when not dieting or weight gain (a benchmark of more than 5% of body weight in a month is suggested); or decrease or increase in appetite nearly every day.

(4) Insomnia or excessive sleep nearly every day.

(5) Psychomotor agitation or retardation nearly every day—as observed by others, not merely subjective.

(6) Fatigue or loss of energy nearly every day.

(7) Feelings of worthlessness, or excessive or inappropriate guilt (which may be delusional) nearly every day.

(8) Reduced ability to think or concentrate or indecisiveness nearly every day.

(9) Recurrent thoughts of death (not just fear of dying), recurrent suicidal ideation without a specific plan, or a suicide attempt or a specific plan for committing suicide.

B. The symptoms lead to significant distress or impairment (e.g. social, occupational).

C. The symptoms are not attributable to the direct effects of a substance (e.g. a drug of abuse, a medication) or a general medical condition.

D. The syndrome is not secondary to a psychotic disorder.

E. There is no history of mania or hypomania unless induced by substances or a medical condition.

Specifiers can be coded for **severity** (mild, moderate, or severe), **psychosis**, and **remission** (partial or full). **Non-coded specifiers** include: anxious distress (see text); whether psychotic symptoms are mood-congruent or mood-incongruent; melancholia (complete anhedonia accompanied by diurnal variation in mood, early morning wakening, total despondency, and psychomotor change); and atypicality (often involving a more reactive mood, hypersomnia, increased appetite, and 'leaden' feelings in the arms or legs).

*For a discussion of the removal of the so-called '***bereavement exclusion***', see Section 5.2.2 and Table 5.4).*

Table 2.1 Classifying depressive disorder		
Classification used in this book	DSM-V (code)	ICD-10 (code)
Major depression	Major depressive episode, single episode, or recurrent (296.21–296.36)	Depressive episode—severe (F32.2), moderate (F32.1), or mild with at least five symptoms (F32.0) Recurrent depressive disorder—current episode severe (F33.2), moderate (F33.1), or mild with at least five symptoms (F33.0)
Sub-threshold depression (includes 'minor' depression)	Other unspecified depressive disorder (311) includes: recurrent brief depression, short-duration depressive episode; and depressive episode with insufficient symptoms Adjustment disorder with depressed mood/mixed anxiety and depressed mood (309.0, 309.28)	Depressive episode—mild with four symptoms (F32.0) Recurrent depressive disorder—current episode mild with four symptoms (F33.0) Mixed anxiety and depressive disorder (F41.2) Adjustment disorder—depressive reaction/mixed anxiety and depressive reaction (F43.2) Other mood (affective) disorders (F38)
	Persistent depressive disorder (dysthymia) (300.4)	Dysthymia (F34.1)

symptoms must be present for at least 2 weeks and are 'pervasive', that is they are there most days, most of the time, and they interfere with the way the person lives his or her life. The syndrome of major depressive episode is defined by criteria A–C.

Another way to look at the syndrome of depression is to look at its impact on the individual. Patients with the syndrome of mild depressive disorder are distressed by their symptoms but can continue to function in life relatively normally. In moderate depression, the individual is more subjectively distressed and can maintain function but with considerable difficulty. Those with severe depression are generally in marked distress and are often agitated or retarded. The ability to function in usual roles is severely limited.

Just because a patient does not meet the diagnostic threshold does not mean their symptoms are unimportant. Having a few symptoms persistently, especially if accompanied by impaired function or quality of life, is a key risk factor for major depression. Often termed sub-threshold depression or minor depression (or dysthymia if chronic), this low-level depression is not trivial since, among the older population, it is associated with adverse health effects, as discussed in the next section. Because sub-syndromal depression in later life is much more common than syndromal depression, its negative impact on the health of the older population is all the greater.

To summarize, depressive disorder is the overall term for any form of depression likely to require, or benefit from, intervention. The two main categories of depressive disorder are major depression and sub-threshold (sub-syndromal) depression. Table 2.1 incorporates some of the other terms that may be encountered and gives the relevant codes from the two major international classificatory systems discussed previously (Anderson *et al.* 2008). ICD-10 and DSM-V differ slightly in that, in ICD-10, only four symptoms are needed to make a diagnosis of depressive episode; this milder form of depression is included under sub-threshold depression.

2.1.1 **Differential diagnosis**

The conditions to consider when interviewing a patient with significant depressive symptoms are shown in Box 2.2.

Depressive disorder is termed 'organic' if there is evidence of a direct link between the onset of depression and either a systemic or neurological condition or an ingested substance or drug. These are coded separately in ICD-10 (F06.31, F06.32) and DSM-V (293.83), although, clinically, they may be indistinguishable from major depression not linked to physical disorder or substance. Causes are discussed in more detail in Chapter 5. Depression accompanying dementia may be classified here, although DSM-V recommends coding both diagnoses if the mood component meets the criteria (see Box 2.1) for a full affective syndrome. Do not forget that alcohol can precipitate or prolong depression.

Bipolar disorder with an onset in later life is infrequent, but recurrent bipolar disorder (from earlier in adulthood) causing bouts of depression is not uncommon. This is known as 'bipolar depression'.

Dysthymia (renamed persistent mood disorder in DSM-V) is a chronic depression with a duration of at least 2 years and a number of symptoms from Box 2.1, although less than that required for major depression. It is often difficult to separate this concept from depressive personality traits or, in older people, the depleting emotional effects of living with chronic handicapping illness. However, persistent mood disorder/dysthymia often has an onset in early life.

In mixed anxiety and depressive disorder, symptoms of depression and anxiety are both present but below the threshold for either depressive episode or generalized anxiety disorder. DSM-V introduces a specifier 'anxious distress'. This may be especially relevant to older patients whose level of anxiety may mask the underlying depression. It comprises feeling tense, restless, worrying, poor concentration, anxious foreboding, and a feeling of impending loss of control.

Lastly, adjustment disorder with depressive reaction is diagnosed when depressive symptoms below the threshold for a diagnosis of depressive episode begin within a month of a serious threat or loss. Symptoms usually resolve within 6 months.

Psychosis can lead to depressive symptoms. Usually, it is clear that the patient's major problem is the presence of delusions and/or hallucinations. By convention, in psychotic conditions, mild to moderate depressive symptoms are considered as secondary to

Box 2.2 Differential diagnosis of depression

Major depressive disorder
Organic depressive disorder
Bipolar affective disorder
Psychotic depression
Dysthymia
Mixed anxiety and depression
Adjustment disorder

the psychosis. A severely depressed patient may present with psychotic symptoms. If due to depression, psychotic experiences are usually 'congruent' that is mood is related to depressive themes of low self-esteem or hopelessness. Occasionally, this is not the case—psychotic symptoms are then termed 'non-congruent'—in which case, the relative importance of the two sets of symptoms, depression and psychosis, must be weighed up. If depression is the more salient symptom, then psychotic depression can be diagnosed, as opposed to as primary psychotic disorder. The particular problem of hypochondriacal delusions is discussed in a later section.

2.2 **Epidemiology**

At all ages, the prevalence of sub-threshold depression significantly exceeds that of major depression. Early research (Kay *et al.* 1964) found that 10% of older adults in the community had what would now correspond to sub-threshold depression (that is significant symptoms but below the threshold for major depression), but only 1.3% met criteria for what we now call major depression. Remarkably similar figures were found in the much more recent EURO-DEP study of depression in later life, conducted in 14 countries—between 8.6 and 14.1% for depressive disorder overall and 1 to 4% for major depression (Copeland *et al.* 1999).

These rates of major depression are lower than those for younger adults. A low rate was also found in the influential North American Epidemiologic Catchment Area (ECA) study (Blazer 2003). Several explanations for the age-related differences in prevalence have been proposed. First, for reasons we do not know, the prevalence of major depression may fall with age. Second, the rates may be underestimates, because studies often exclude individuals in care homes where the prevalence of depression is high. Excluding people with depressive symptoms soon after bereavement from being diagnosed with depressive disorder is likely to disproportionately affect rates of diagnosis in older people. The strict checklist approach of DSM and ICD to diagnosing major depression may not be suited to older populations. There is some evidence for this. Prince *et al.* (1999) used an age-specific depression scale 'EURO-D' to compare symptoms of depression among older adults in Europe. Two factors encapsulated the majority of depressive symptoms. One was 'affective suffering' (characterized by depression, tearfulness, and a wish to die), and the other was a 'motivation' factor (comprising loss of interest, poor concentration, and lack of enjoyment). The motivation factor increased with age, whereas affective suffering remained the same across age groups. The constellation of symptoms suggested by the motivation factor does not fit readily with ICD or DSM. This factor may, therefore, be specific to later life, meaning that, rather than falling in later life, the prevalence of depressive disorder may increase when co-morbidity from depleting medical conditions is factored in.

Medical co-morbidity and cognitive impairment are the two key factors which affect the diagnosis and management of depressive disorder in older adults. Because of this, rates of depression (including major depression) in long-term care facilities, such as residential and nursing homes, are typically up to three times higher than among community residents (Blazer 2003). The combination of physical frailty and cognitive impairment results in even higher rates.

A similar picture is seen among older patients admitted to the medical and surgical wards of acute hospitals, with rates averaging 10–12% for major depression (Blazer

2003). Cognitive impairment is also associated with high rates of depression, upward of 17% for Alzheimer's disease and even higher for vascular and subcortical dementias (Alexopoulos 2005).

Is age itself a risk factor for depression? In a large cohort study, Robert *et al.* (1997) found that **healthy** older people were not at greater risk of depression than younger ones. Higher prevalence with age was explained by the poorer health of the older subjects, rather than their age.

2.3 **Impact of depression**

In 1990, it was estimated that mental and neurological disorders accounted for 10% of the total disability adjusted life years (DALYs) lost due to all diseases and injuries. In 2000, this rose to 12%. By 2020, it is projected that the burden of these disorders, among all age groups, will have increased to 15% (World Health Organization 2001). Contained within this report, the Global Burden of Disease study (GBD 2000) indicated that unipolar depressive disorders accounted for 4.4% of the global disease burden, the fourth most disabling disorder after respiratory conditions, perinatal conditions, and HIV/AIDS and ahead of diarrhoeal diseases, ischaemic heart disease, and cerebrovascular disease.

Sub-threshold depression is associated with functional impairment approaching that of major depression (Blazer 2003). Risk factors for sub-threshold depression (minor depression) in later life are similar to those for major depression (see Chapter 5). Minor (sub-threshold) depression is also a risk factor for major depressive episode. Given the scale of sub-threshold depression, it alone adds substantially considerably to the burden due to depression.

Key references

Alexopoulos GS (2005). Depression in the elderly. *The Lancet*, **365**, 1961–70.

American Psychiatric Association (APA) (2013). *Diagnostic and Statistical Manual Version V*. American Psychiatric Association, Washington DC.

Anderson IM, Ferrier IN, Baldwin R, *et al.*; on behalf of the Consensus Meeting; endorsed by the British Association for Psychopharmacology Evidence (2008). Evidence-based guidelines for treating depressive disorders with antidepressants: a revision of the 2000 British Association for Psychopharmacology guidelines. *Journal of Psychopharmacology*, **22**, 343–96.

Blazer DG (2003). Depression in late life: review and commentary. *Journal of Gerontology: Medical Sciences*, **58A**, 249–65.

Copeland JRM, Beekman ATF, Dewey ME, *et al.* (1999). Depression in Europe: geographical distribution among older people. *British Journal of Psychiatry*, **174**, 312–21.

Kay DW, Beamish P, Roth M (1964). Old age mental disorders in Newcastle-Upon-Tyne, Part I: a study of prevalence. *British Journal of Psychiatry*, **110**, 146–58.

National Institute for Health and Clinical Excellence (2009). *NICE clinical guideline 90 Depression: the treatment and management of depression in adults (partial update of NICE clinical guideline 23)*. National Institute for Health and Clinical Excellence, London.

Paykel ES and Priest RG (1992). Recognition and management of depression in general practice: consensus statement. *BMJ*, **305**, 1198–202.

Prince MJ, Beekman ATF, Deeg DJH, *et al.* (1999). Depression symptoms in late life assessed using the EURO-D scale: effect of age, gender and marital status in 14 European centres. *British Journal of Psychiatry*, **174**, 339–45.

Robert RE, Kaplan GA, Shema SJ, Strawbridge WJ (1997). Does growing old increase the risk for depression? *American Journal of Psychiatry*, **154**, 1384–90.

World Health Organization (1994). *The ICD-10 classification of mental and behavioural disorders*. World Health Organization, Geneva.

World Health Organization (2001). *The world health report 2001—mental health: new understanding, new hope*. World Health Organization, Geneva.

Chapter 3

Clinical features

Key points

- Two main differences in the presentation of late-life depression are that a complaint of depression may be minimized and somatic concern (hypochondriasis) is present.
- Apathy and depression differ, and the former is often associated with executive cognitive problems and vascular brain disease.
- Cognitive impairment is common in late-life depression and is often irreversible.

3.1 Symptoms

3.1.1 Key age-related factors

Brodaty *et al.* (2001) examined the effect of age of onset on the phenomenology of late-life depression in 810 patients referred to a tertiary mood disorders service in Australia. Some clinical types, such psychotic depression, and some clinical features, such as psychomotor agitation or retardation, marked withdrawal, hypochondriasis, and severe guilt, were more common in older patients and were associated more with age than with age at onset, an effect more pronounced in females. In this study, subjective reports of depressed mood were lower in older patients, whereas objective measures were higher. This disparity increased markedly with age and supports the view that older patients minimize feelings of sadness.

Taken together, data like these suggest that there are two key features that distinguish late-life depressive disorders in older people: when depressed, they complain less of sadness than younger adults, and they often become excessively concerned about physical health (somatic concern or hypochondriasis). Depression without sadness is not the contradiction that it sounds, because, on more detailed interview, there will invariably be other symptoms of depressive disorder (see Box 2.1); the problem is that these two key features can obscure the diagnosis of depression.

Why these changes in the presentation of depression in later life occur is a matter of speculation, but generational differences probably play a large part. Those who grew up after the austerity which followed the World Wars learned to be stoic and to 'not bother the doctor' with emotional difficulties. As children, the observance of a regular bowel habit was probably more ingrained than it is today, which might explain why the bowel becomes such a frequent preoccupation among older people when depressed.

A point to be aware of is that there is sometimes a 'disconnect' between the older person's medical history and their hypochondriacal complaints when depressed. For example, a patient may have good reason to be concerned about their heart if they suffer from ischaemic heart disease causing breathlessness and angina. When depressed, (s)he may present with heightened anxiety and preoccupation about the heart but might just as easily start to become preoccupied with unrelated concerns, for example, fear of bowel blockage, even though there is no medical history of bowel disease. We do not know what dictates which scenario the patient may follow, but both can lead to mistakes. In the first scenario, the practitioner may go on a 'wild goose chase', looking for evidence of a worsened cardiac state and overlooking the depressive disorder causing the increased cardiac concern. Equally, in the second scenario, speculative investigations may be undertaken in an attempt to link known pathology to the new presentation, again missing depression as the cause of the 'disconnect'. However, there **is** a need to conduct appropriate investigation of newly presenting depressive disorder, and this will be considered in Chapter 6.

3.1.2 **Psychosis**

Although there is some debate as to whether psychotic (delusional) symptoms in depression simply reflect a more severe form of depression or that psychotic depression is a specific subtype, there does seem to be a higher likelihood of psychosis occurring in late-life depression. The classical delusions of depression include guilt, poverty, and worthlessness, but, in older age, hypochondriacal delusions are often prominent (Baldwin 1995). Another psychotic presentation is Cotard's syndrome, in which patients may negate their own body or their existence. For example, a severely depressed patient once dismissed the author, saying there was no point in any questions as she was already dead and was awaiting the ambulance to take her body away. Abnormal perceptions, such as auditory hallucinations, may also occur in severe depression. Usually, these take the form of a voice in the third person making derogatory remarks. The content is often 'congruent' with the mood (for example, 'you're worthless' in someone with very negative views of self). Box 3.1 illustrates some vignettes.

Sometimes, detecting psychotic beliefs can be difficult in profoundly withdrawn patients. It is one of the factors to consider in patients with treatment-resistant depression, as depression with psychotic symptoms rarely responds to an antidepressant alone. This is discussed further in Chapter 7, but clues include a past history of this presentation (as psychosis in depression tends to 'run true'), frequent muttering or distraction as if responding to internal or external stimuli, oppositional behaviour suggesting persecutory ideation (for example, believing food is poisoned and so refusing it), and escalating requests for medical help regarding specific symptoms which have already been addressed.

3.1.3 **Apathy and amotivation**

Apathy (literally, a loss of 'pathos') is generally defined as a lack of goal-directed activity or thought and/or a lack of goal-related emotional response. Often, it is summarized as 'the spark is missing' (van Reekum *et al.* 2005). As a disorder of motivation, rather than mood, apathy is distinct from depression. Like depression, apathy is used either to denote a symptom or a syndrome. The syndromal aspects may be experienced in

Box 3.1 Vignettes (hypochondriacal presentations of depression)

A 75-year-old man was admitted to hospital after cutting his wrist. He was clearly depressed, but, after 6 weeks' treatment with an antidepressant, there was little improvement. His lack of reassurance about his health (which was good), increasing requests to see 'the chief doctor', and the uncovering of an earlier history of profound weight loss, eventually diagnosed as depression, made the treating team suspect delusions. Eventually, he confessed to an unshakeable belief that he had syphilis. A negative test briefly reassured him, but his delusion only left after introducing an antipsychotic drug. The final diagnosis was psychotic depression.

An 86-year-old woman of anxious disposition presented to her primary care physician 3 weeks after seeing her hairdresser, whom she believed may have accidentally introduced 'some sort of infection' via hair curlers. Despite reassurance, she presented serially with complaints that her scalp was itchy and that her cheeks were 'on fire', preventing her from sleeping. Realizing that this must be a psychological complaint, the physician uncovered low mood, marked morning anxiety, early morning waking, and decreased function. Moderate non-psychotic depressive disorder was diagnosed, caused by recent worries about her husband's ill health.

the affective, behavioural, or cognitive domains, resulting in indifference, indolence, and impoverished thoughts, respectively. It is associated with stroke, traumatic brain injury, frontal lobe degeneration, degenerative dementias, multiple sclerosis as well as depressive disorder (Van Reekum *et al.* 2005). It is particularly seen in basal ganglia diseases and conditions which disrupt the integrity of the subcortical-frontal connections, especially involving the anterior cingulate and the dorsolateral pre-frontal cortex. Together, these are known as fronto-striatal circuits (FSC). FSC are important in late-life depression, as any disruption causes a 'dysexecutive syndrome', a cognitive syndrome which will be discussed in the next section.

Apathy is not the same as depression, although there is overlap and both may lead to low interest and effort. How can the two be distinguished? As shown in Figure 3.1, depressive disorder is a disorder of mood which often has secondary effects on motivation and is experienced as highly distressing for the individual. Apathy is primarily a disorder of motivation which decreases subjective response, including distress, which is, therefore, felt more by caregivers. Box 3.2 offers a vignette. Depression responds to psychological treatments and medication whilst apathy may require a behavioural intervention.

3.1.4 **Typical presentations**

Although there are few symptoms which incontrovertibly distinguish late-life from early-onset depression, there are differences in clinical presentation. As discussed, a complaint of depression is understated among older people and may be attributed to physical illness, although there is, of course, a significant overlap of some depressive symptoms with some symptoms of physical illness (for example, poor appetite). These considerations may accentuate some aspects of presentation whilst other factors tend to obscure the diagnosis (see Box 3.3).

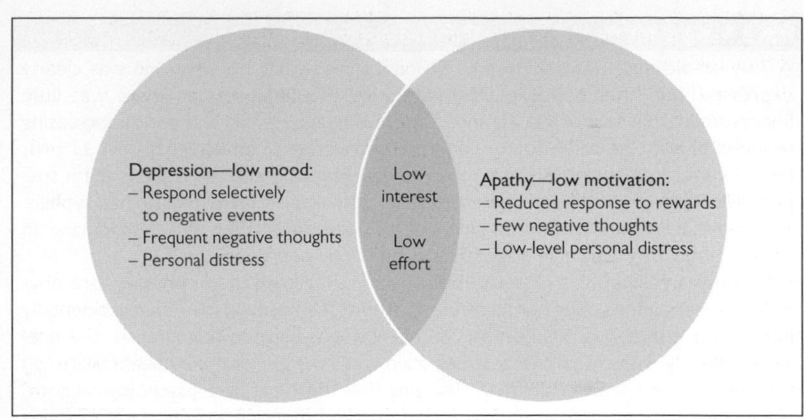

Figure 3.1 The overlap between depression and apathy.

Box 3.2 Apathy and depression

A 68-year-old man presented with food refusal and an insidious 10 kg weight loss. His wife had died a year earlier, and impaired mobility had led to an admission to a nursing home, during which time the weight loss had occurred. Staff brought food to his room but were usually dismissed with a curt remark about not being bothered with food, although, sometimes if they left food, it would be eaten. Lately, instead of merely declining food, he became hostile and swore; his sleep was disrupted, and he reported having a lot more back pain. He was admitted to the psychiatric unit where moderate depressive disorder was diagnosed, and investigations revealed multiple degenerative vertebral disc fractures. His apathy and disinhibited behaviour suggested frontal lobe impairment, confirmed on neuropsychological testing and probably due to past heavy drinking. Treatment comprised antidepressant and improved analgesia. His mood and irritability improved, but his apathy regarding food required the introduction of a structured behavioural programme aimed at reinforcing pleasurable aspects of eating and discouraging eating alone in his room. With this, his weight increased.

A frequent difficulty is the overlap of depression with co-morbid medical illness. DSM takes an aetiological approach to mood symptoms, meaning that the clinician must judge whether a symptom (for example, reduced appetite) is due to physical illness and, if so, discount it in diagnosing depression. An alternative inclusive approach makes no aetiological assumptions and counts all symptoms, whether or not better explained by co-morbid illnesses. Koenig *et al.* (1997) applied a range of strategies from the purely aetiological approach to an inclusive one and showed, not surprisingly, that they resulted in a twofold difference in the assessed prevalence of major depression.

Take the following example. An individual with active rheumatoid arthritis may experience insomnia, fatigue, and poor appetite equally from his or her physical illness or an associated depression. For a practitioner with little experience in mental health, the

Box 3.3 Important aspects of the clinical presentation of late-life depression

Minimal expression of sadness
Somatization or excessive physical (hypochondriacal) complaints
Overlap of physical and somatic psychiatric symptoms
Unexplained pain syndromes
Neurotic symptoms of recent onset
Medically 'trivial' acts of deliberate self-harm
'Pseudodementia'
Depression superimposed upon dementia
Accentuation of abnormal personality traits
Behaviour disorder
Late-onset alcohol dependency syndrome
'Loneliness'
Insomnia

inclusive approach will probably be safest but may result in over-diagnosing depression. A more experienced practitioner will be able to make a judgement about the likelihood of this symptom being more likely to be due to depression or medical co-morbidity. The history is pivotal. For example, early morning wakening may emerge from a background of more generalized sleep disturbance due to pain. Questions must be appropriate. For example, for those with limited mobility or exercise tolerance, a question such as 'Do you feel tired even when resting?' is preferable to 'Have you no energy?'. With the patient's permission, a history from someone close is often informative. It is important to ascertain whether there has been any prior history of depression, which may increase the likelihood of the current symptoms being due to depression.

There is growing awareness that depression may present predominantly with pain. The pain is often non-specific. Headache, abdominal pain, or musculoskeletal pains in the lower back, joints, and neck are common and may occur in combination so that the clinician should have a high index of suspicion in patients presenting with multiple pain symptoms of unclear aetiology. 'Pain all over' can be a culturally determined presentation in some parts of the world, for example, south Asia.

So-called neurotic symptoms of recent onset in later life should not be taken at face value. The sudden occurrence of marked anxiety, obsessional compulsive phenomena, hysteria, or hypochondriasis in an older person not previously neurotically prone should serve as a prompt to look closely for depressive disorder, which is the usual cause. Likewise, at all levels of severity of depression, anxiety is a common accompanying symptom. If it dominates the clinical picture, it may mask the depressive disorder.

'Pseudodementia' has been used in several different ways but, most characteristically, when an older patient presents with vociferous complaints of poor memory, many 'don't know' responses, and a relatively recent onset. Although these patients appear to be amnesic with poor attention, they do not have deficits in higher cortical function, such as aphasia, agraphia, or acalculia which characterize dementia. Pseudodementia is a term which has probably outlived its usefulness. Other terms, such as 'dementia of depression' (Pearlson *et al.* 1989) or 'depression-executive dysfunction syndrome' (Alexopoulos *et al.* 2002) are now used (see Section 3.2).

Less discussed in the literature, but readily recognizable to clinicians working with older patients, is when depression shows itself under the guise of a disorder of behaviour. Presentations with food refusal, 'incontinence' (for example, a perverse ability to eliminate in almost any place other than the toilet, unlike the incontinence of dementia), screaming, and outwardly aggressive behaviour may occur, often in a residential or nursing home facility where the person is resentful of having been admitted. A history from someone who knows the patient is crucial. This will often highlight a recent change in mood and vitality.

The advent of depressive disorder may lead to an accentuation of pre-morbid personality traits. A previously anxious and dependant person when depressed may present with theatricality and ceaseless importuning, sometimes to several agencies simultaneously, for example, social services, primary care, and the local accident and emergency department. Other behavioural problems which may occur indicating an underlying depressive disorder in older people include shoplifting in a hitherto honest person.

Late-onset alcohol dependence syndrome is a recognized complication of depression and a mode of presentation of depression. In later life, there are two types of alcohol-dependent individuals: those who have drunk heavily from a younger age (so-called 'survivors'), for whom the systemic adverse effects of alcohol (liver, cardiac, brain) exert an increasing toll; and those who commence drinking in later life in response to loneliness, grief, or, not infrequently, depressive disorder. There is growing evidence that, if detected, this kind of damaging drinking can be helped considerably by targeted treatment of the alcohol dependency as well as treatment of depression (IAS 2010).

A complaint of loneliness from an individual who previously coped quite well alone, often accompanied by a request to be re-housed, should raise a suspicion of depressive disorder.

There is a complex relationship between insomnia and depression. It is both a symptom, which heralds depression, and a risk factor for it. Because insomnia occurs more frequently with age, it can too readily be dismissed as 'ageing'. Again, a good history can elucidate a change in the quality of poor sleep.

3.2 Cognitive disturbance in depression

3.2.1 The nature and significance of cognitive impairment in late-life depression

Many patients with late-life major depression have cognitive impairment. It is now recognized that this frequently persists after treatment, probably due to the combined effect of depression and age-related brain changes, such as atrophy and vascular disease.

The speed of information processing is impaired in depressive disorder, notably on tasks requiring sustained effort. Poor memory associated with depression usually improves with cueing, whereas, in dementia, it does not. This is because the earliest (registration) stage of memory is affected in dementia so that the information is not merely difficult to access but non-existent. Functional imaging suggests that the areas of the brain involved in the cognitive disorder of Alzheimer's disease are different from those involved in the cognitive impairment seen in major depression (Dolan *et al.* 1992). However, amnesia and depression can be early symptoms of Alzheimer's disease whilst, in chronic depression, hypercortisolaemia due to dysregulation of the hypo-pituitary-adrenal axis (HPA) may cause subtle hippocampal damage, leading to memory impairment.

Deficits in higher-order cognition are not usually affected by depression alone, rather there are deficits in executive tasks (planning, initiation, and task persistence) and speed of information processing (Butters *et al.* 2004). The is the depression-executive dysfunction syndrome (DEDS) in late-life depression (Alexopoulos *et al.* 2002), mentioned earlier in connection with 'pseudodementia'. Clinically, these patients present with slow inefficient thinking and patchy memory impairment and are often apathetic. Some authorities regard executive problems as a particular feature of late-onset major depression, whereas older people with early-onset depression may experience more specific memory disturbance. This also implies different aetiological pathways: executive dysfunction arising from vascular injury to the FSC and amnesia from neurodegeneration of the hippocampus, but this is not proven.

3.2.2 **Differentiating depression from dementia**

This important differential diagnosis starts with the history (see Table 3.1). Dementia usually begins and proceeds slowly, compared to major depression. Typically, in dementia, relatives and caregivers are the first to notice memory problems, whereas, in depression, it is usually the patient who complains of a 'bad' memory. On memory testing, those with dementia may guess answers whilst patients with depression may struggle to summon the effort and simply give up with an 'I don't know'. As discussed, this reflects too the fact that dementia affects higher cortical function, such as higher-order memory, whereas depressive disorder affects concentration and information processing, often referred to as 'subcortical'.

Given the importance of making the correct diagnosis, Olin *et al.* (2002) have proposed criteria for the diagnosis of depression in Alzheimer's disease. Their criteria emphasize symptoms, such as reduced positive affect, social isolation, and withdrawal (see Box 3.4). Another useful avenue is screening, and the Cornell scale (see Appendix) was devised to detect depressive disorder in dementia.

Table 3.1 Dementia and depression

Dementia	Depression
Insidious	Rapid onset
Symptoms usually of long duration	Symptoms usually of short duration
Mood and behaviour fluctuate	Mood is consistently depressed
'Near miss' answers typical	'Don't know' answers typical
Patient conceals forgetfulness	Patient highlights forgetfulness
Cognitive impairment relatively stable	Cognitive impairment fluctuates greatly
Higher cortical dysfunction evident	Higher cortical dysfunction absent

Box 3.4 Provisional criteria for depression in Alzheimer's disease

A. Three (or more) of the following symptoms have been present during the same 2-week period and represent a change from previous functioning: at least one of the symptoms is either (1) depressed mood or (2) decreased positive affect or pleasure.

Note: do not include symptoms that, in your judgement, are clearly due to a medical condition other than Alzheimer's disease or are a direct result of non-mood-related dementia symptoms (e.g. loss of weight due to difficulties with food intake).

1) Clinically significant depressed mood (e.g. depressed, sad, hopeless, discouraged, tearful).
2) Decreased positive affect or pleasure in response to social contacts and usual activities.
3) Social isolation or withdrawal.
4) Disruption in appetite.
5) Disruption in sleep.
6) Psychomotor changes (e.g. agitation or retardation).
7) Irritability.
8) Fatigue or loss of energy.
9) Feelings of worthlessness, hopelessness, or excessive or inappropriate guilt.
10) Recurrent thoughts of death, suicidal ideation, plan, or attempt.

B. All criteria are met for dementia of the Alzheimer's type.

C. The symptoms cause clinically significant distress or disruption in functioning.

D. The symptoms do not occur exclusively during the course of a delirium.

E. The symptoms are not due to the direct physiological effects of a substance (e.g. a drug of abuse or a medication).

F. The symptoms are not better accounted for by other conditions, such as a major depressive disorder, bipolar disorder, bereavement, schizophrenia, schizoaffective disorder, psychosis of Alzheimer's disease, anxiety disorders, or substance-related disorder.

Adapted from The American Journal of Geriatric Psychiatry, Volume 10, Issue 2, Olin, Jason T. et al, Provisional Diagnostic Criteria for Depression of Alzheimer Disease, 125–128, Copyright (2002), with permission from Elsevier.

3.2.3 **Depression occurring during established cognitive impairment and dementia**

Between 30–50% of people with Alzheimer's disease have significant depressive symptoms, as do a quarter of those with precursor states, such as mild cognitive impairment (MCI) (Potter and Steffens 2007).

Key references

Alexopoulos GS, Kiosses DN, Klimstra S, Kalayam B, Bruce ML (2002). Clinical presentation of the 'depression-executive dysfunction syndrome' of late life. *American Journal of Geriatric Psychiatry*, **10**, 98–106.

Baldwin RC (1995). Delusional depression in elderly patients: characteristics and relationship to age at onset. *International Journal of Geriatric Psychiatry*, **10**, 981–5.

Brodaty H, Luscombe G, Parker G, *et al.* (2001). Early and late onset depression in old age: different aetiologies, same phenomenology. *Journal of Affective Disorders*, **66**, 225–36.

Butters MA, Whyte EM, Nebes RD, *et al.* (2004). The nature and determinants of neuropsychological functioning in late-life depression. *Archives of General Psychiatry*, **61**, 587–95.

Dolan RJ, Bench CJ, Brown RG, Scott LC, Friston KJ, Frackowiak RSJ (1992). Regional cerebral blood flow abnormalities in depressed patients with cognitive impairment. *Journal of Neurology, Neurosurgery and Psychiatry*, **55**, 768–73.

Institute of Alcohol Studies (IAS) (2010). *Alcohol and the elderly.* IAS Factsheet, Cambs. (downloadable from <http://www.ias.org.uk/Alcohol-knowledge-centre/Alcohol-and-older-people.aspx>)

Koenig HG, George LK, Peterson BL, Pieper CF (1997). Depression in medically ill hospitalized older adults: prevalence, characteristics, and course of symptoms according to six diagnostic schemes. *American Journal of Psychiatry*, **154**, 1376–83.

Olin JT, Schneider LS, Katz IR, *et al.* (2002). Provisional diagnostic criteria for depression of Alzheimer disease. *American Journal of Geriatric Psychiatry*, **10**, 125–8.

Pearlson GD, Rabins PV, Kim WS, *et al.* (1989). Structural brain CT changes and cognitive deficits with and without reversible dementia ('pseudodementia'). *Psychological Medicine*, **19**, 573–84.

Potter GG and Steffens DC (2007). Contribution of depression to cognitive impairment and dementia in older adults. *The Neurologist*, **13**, 105–17.

Van Reekum R, Stuss DT, Ostrander L (2005). Apathy: why care? *Journal of Neuropsychiatry and Clinical Neurosciences*, **17**, 7–19.

Chapter 4

Self-harm and suicide

Key points

- Suicide is over-represented in older, compared to younger, populations.
- The clinical characteristics of those who self-harm in later life closely resemble those of completed suicides.
- Beware of the 'medically trivial' overdose or other act of self-harm in an older person; mostly, this will reflect a serious attempt.
- Suicide prevention should focus on recognition and treatment of depression, particularly in primary care.

In many countries where there are reliable data, suicide rates are highest among older adults. In the United States, from 1980 to 1992, the suicide rate among the over 65s rose by 9%, but, among those aged 80–84, it increased by 35%. Some trends are surprising. For example, in a UK survey of the south Asian population, the highest rate was amongst women aged over 65 (McKenzie *et al.* 2008).

Attempted suicide in older adults closely resembles successful suicide in its clinical characteristics. A (literally) fatal mistake then is not to take seriously an act of deliberate self-harm because it appears to be medically trivial. Elderly people rarely take overdoses merely to draw attention, to resolve tension, or merely by accident. Most have depressive disorder, and all require a psychiatric assessment. More difficult to characterize is the concept of depression presenting as 'sub-intentional' suicide. This might be suspected in individuals who are profoundly withdrawn, reject assistance, refuse food, and suffer severe weight loss. However, patients who 'turn their face to the wall' are a heterogeneous group, some of whom may be severely depressed, but others turn out to have undiagnosed medical problems, such as carcinoma.

It is clearly important to recognize older people at high risk of suicide. Previous self-harm is the factor most predictive of later suicide. Several other factors add to the risk. Box 4.1 lists them under three headings: general factors in the community, features of the depression, and specific behaviours. The means of suicide in older people varies from culture to culture. Overdose, especially of benzodiazepines and non-opiate analgesics, is common in Western cultures, but, in the United States, firearm use by older men is becoming more frequent.

Suicide is sometimes viewed as a failure of specialist psychiatric services. In reality, most older people who kill themselves are not patients of psychiatric services. Of those who do go on to end their lives, a majority have had contact with primary care services, so vigilance in primary care is vital for any preventive approach to be successful.

Box 4.1 Suicide risk in later life

General factors

Any past suicide attempt or episode of self-harm
Male gender
Living alone
Inadequate social support
Life events involving loss (for example, bereavement) and negative events
Chronic stressors (for example, environmental or financial)
Chronic medical conditions, including cancer (especially if painful)
Alcohol misuse
Rigid personality styles
Cultural acceptability (in some societies, suicide is more acceptable than in others)

Illness factors

Mental disorder (any mood disorder, psychosis, or substance misuse)
Agitation
Insomnia
Guilt
Hopelessness
Low self-esteem
Hypochondriacal preoccupations

Specific behaviours

Suicide intent or plans expressed
'Accidental' overdose
Leaving notes for those left behind
Altering wills
Hoarding tablets
Severe self-neglect

Primary care practitioners should take seriously statements concerning self-harm and try to remove a means of carrying out the act in those about whom they have concerns. It is important to be alert to behaviours, such as suddenly altering wills, giving away possessions, or sudden changes in religious interest. Although they exist, over-reliance on suicide rating scales is unwise. The use of a relatively impersonal suicide rating questionnaire in someone who requires immense empathy might make matters worse. If in doubt, patients should undergo a specialist assessment.

Suicide prevention programmes have been developed in a number of countries, often deploying a broad strategic approach with an emphasis on detection and treatment of depression. In Hong Kong, five suicide prevention teams, aimed at older adults, were established. These comprised psychiatrists, nurses, and social workers (Chiu *et al.* 2003). The teams work collaboratively with telephone support services, non-governmental organizations, centres for the elderly, and general practitioners (GPs) to screen for depression and identify those at risk of suicide. Older people with suicidal risk or who are severely depressed are seen in fast-track clinics and visited at home by nurses, with ongoing telephone monitoring. Other initiatives focus on the provision of training for GPs in the detection and management of depression and collaborative care models of risk reduction (see Section 8.5). One such programme, the Prevention of Suicide in Primary Care Elderly: Collaborative Trial (PROSPECT), found that, among those identified with milder forms of depression, the intervention reduced suicidal ideation (Bruce *et al.* 2004). An intervention which prevents the development of suicidal thinking at an early stage is an attractive one.

There are factors which can reduce suicidal risk. Given that pain and disability are associated with suicide, effective management of physical illness and control of pain may help to reduce this. In the UK, the suicide rate among elderly people fell after replacing coal gas with non-noxious natural gas, suggesting that removing a means of suicide may help prevention. Personal resilience is important—developing or regaining a sense of meaning and purpose in life is protective, as is religious practice.

Key references

Bruce ML, Have TRT, Reynolds CF, *et al.* (2004). Reducing suicidal ideation and depressive symptoms in depressed older primary care patients: a randomized controlled trial. *Journal of the American Medical Association*, **291**, 1081–91.

Chiu HFK, Takahashi H, Suh GH (2003). Elderly suicide prevention in East Asia. *International Journal of Geriatric Psychiatry*, **18**, 973–6.

McKenzie K, Bhui K, Nanchahal K, Blizard B (2008). Suicide rates in people of South Asian origin in England and Wales: 1993–2003. *British Journal of Psychiatry*, **193**, 406–9.

Chapter 5

Aetiology

Key points
• Disability and handicap are closely linked to the aetiology of late-life depressive disorder. • Always check for underlying physical illness and various prescribed drugs as potential causes of depressive disorder in later life. • Vascular disease (vascular depression) is increasingly recognized as a cause of late-onset depressive disorder. • However, in many cases of late-life depression, the cause is multifactorial. • Being a caregiver of someone with dementia is associated with a high risk of depression.

Often, there are multiple causes and pathways to depressive disorder in later life (see vignette in Box 5.1) and often an overlap of co-morbidities, such as physical disease, cognitive impairment, and alcohol misuse. To aid thinking, the aetiology can be subdivided into the three 'p's: predisposing risk factors, precipitating factors, and perpetuating features (see Table 5.1). A fourth 'p' acts as a reminder that patients also have factors which protect against depression and can be deployed in management.

5.1 Predisposing factors

5.1.1 Genetic susceptibility

There is less genetic susceptibility to depression in later, than younger, life. An exception is depressive episode occurring as part of bipolar affective disorder, which often recurs into later life and has a strong genetic basis. In contrast to its role in dementia, no definite role has been established for the ε4 allele of the apolipoprotein E gene in the origin of late-life depression.

5.1.2 Gender and civil status

At all ages, depression is more frequent in women, especially in widows and divorcees.

5.1.3 Past psychiatric history

A history of depressive disorder or dysthymia in earlier life is an undoubted risk factor for late-life depression (Cole and Dendukuri 2003). Alcohol dependency and schizophrenia are associated with depression.

Box 5.1 Vignette to illustrate aetiological factors

Mr M is 74 and has been asked to come in by his primary care practice for a scheduled blood pressure and diabetes review. The practice nurse notes that, although his clothes are reasonably smart, they are loose and there is a smell of stale urine. His movements are slow and his speech hesitant and mumbling. When answering questions, he looks into his hands which he is wringing. After a review of his blood pressure, diabetes, and medication, Mr M asks for something to help with his sleep. The nurse notes on his last visit a year ago that his wife was very ill, and now Mr M states tearfully that she died 4 months ago. On further questioning, he reports losing his appetite. Thoughts about his wife keep him awake in bed at night. He has lost interest in reading and mixing with his friends at the pub, and he states he is embarrassed to admit to his friends that he drinks three pints of beer and two large whiskies at night on his own. Increasingly, over the past month, he has dwelt on pessimistic thoughts and feelings that he should have seen signs that his wife was going to have a stroke. In the night, he has thought about how much better it would be if he did not wake up and has sometimes wished he were dead so that he can join his wife, although he has never thought of harming himself. Sometimes, he forgets what day it is and last week missed an appointment with the optician. He has two children, but they are over 100 miles away. He has always regarded himself as a worrier. In his medical history, he had coronary bypass surgery 2 years ago. Two months ago, he had a short admission to hospital for heart failure, for which he was given a beta-blocker which helped his breathing. Mr M agrees that the nurse can discuss his problem with his GP to confirm whether this might be depression. Later, the nurse meets the GP in a practice meeting, and Dr P remembers that Mr M was seen for depression about 6 years ago after his wife had a mild stroke.

Mr M displays many typical aetiological factors in late-life depression, and the case shows how these often occur together, cumulatively adding to the risk of becoming depressed. He is predisposed to depression because he has had it in the past, depression being an inherently recurrent disorder. Diabetes is a known risk factor for depression as well as vascular disease which, along with his hypertension, may predispose him to vascular depression, characterized by slowed thoughts and patchy memory loss (see Section 5.4.4). The same factors can also predispose to dementia which too is a risk factor for depression. Coronary artery disease is associated with a twofold increase in the chances of depression. Social isolation and loneliness are recognized risk factors for depression. Some personality traits are associated with depression, notably anxious, dependent, and obsessional. His bereavement is a major trigger for his depression. Possibly too is the relatively recent introduction of a beta-blocker, and all medication should be reviewed from the perspective of possible depressogenic effects. Last, increased alcohol consumption is not uncommon in late-onset depression, and continued heavy driving can exacerbate and/or perpetuate depressive symptoms.

5.1.4 **Physical ill health, impairment, and handicap**

The interaction between ill health and depressive disorders is complex and bidirectional; chronic ill health can predispose to depression as well as worsening its prognosis, and the presence of a depressive disorder can also worsen the outcome of

Table 5.1 Factors involved in the causation of late-life depression			
Predisposing	**Precipitating**	**Perpetuating**	**Protective**
Genes (minimal)	Adverse life events (usually of loss)	Poor health	Adaptive coping style
Gender and civil status	Chronic stress and difficulties	Social adversity	Resilience
Past psychiatric history	Medication	Handicap	Affiliation (e.g. religious group)
Physical ill health, impairment, and handicap		Poor social support	High level of perceived support
Sensory impairment		Relationship and family difficulties	Positive life events
Personality (avoidant, dependent, obsessional)			
Psychosocial (poverty, crime, and loneliness)			
Degree of acculturation			
Caregiving			

physical illness. A vicious cycle may establish itself, in which physical impairment provokes depression, which may, in turn, add to the disability of the underlying impairment (Prince *et al*. 1998).

Other factors associated with ageing, such as hearing and visual loss, predispose to depressive disorder (Rovner *et al*. 2007). Also, frequent primary care attendance and a high level of home support are possible markers for depressive disorder (Katona and Shankar 2004).

Ischaemic heart disease, several neurological disorders (such as Parkinson's disease and Alzheimer's disease), cerebrovascular disease (such as vascular dementia and stroke), hip fracture, and chronic obstructive pulmonary disease have all been associated with a high rate of depression in older adults (Alexopoulos 2005; Blazer 2003). Pain syndromes of various causes are also closely linked to depression. Again, these associations are bidirectional: depression worsens pain, and pain leads to depression. A range of disorders, some not obvious at presentation, can predispose to depressive disorder (see Table 5.2). Co-morbidity is considered in more detail in Chapter 6.

There are several mechanisms whereby medical conditions may lead to depression. For the neurological disorders, such as the dementias, stroke, and Parkinson's disease, alteration in the brain serotonergic systems may be important. However, the wide range of disabling medical conditions which seem to increase vulnerability to depression suggests that the meaning of the illness for the sufferer is as important as the precise organ system involved. Prince *et al*. (1998) have shown that the concept of handicap—the disadvantage in society resulting from impairment and disability—is an important risk factor for depression in older people. This concept not only helps to understand depression but emphasizes that handicap is as much a societal issue as a medical one. Two older people may be similarly impaired by medical illnesses, but, if

Table 5.2 Medical conditions and central-acting drugs that may cause organic depressive disorder	
Medical conditions	**Central-acting drugs**
Endocrine/metabolic	**Antihypertensive drugs**
Hypo/hyperthyroidism	Beta-blockers (especially non-selective)
Cushing's disease	Methyldopa
Hypercalcaemia	Reserpine
Sub-nutrition	Clonidine
Pernicious anaemia	Nifedipine, calcium channel agents
Organic brain disease	Digoxin
Cerebrovascular disease/stroke	**Steroids**
CNS tumours	**Analgesic drugs**
Parkinson's disease	Opioids
Alzheimer's disease and vascular dementia	Indometacin
Multiple sclerosis	**Anti-Parkinson's**
Systemic lupus erythematosus	Levodopa
Occult carcinoma	Amantadine
Pancreas	Tetrabenazine
Lung	**Psychiatric drugs**
Chronic infections	Neuroleptics
Neurosyphilis	Benzodiazepines
Brucellosis	**Miscellaneous**
Neurocysticercosis	Sulfonamides
Myalgic encephalomyelitis	Alcohol
HIV	Interferon

one has limited practical support and poor access to transport, she is the more handicapped. The implications for treating depression are obvious.

5.1.5 **Personality and developmental factors**

Structured personality assessment suggests that personality dysfunction, especially of the 'avoidant' and 'dependent' types, is associated with late-life depression (Blazer and Hybels 2005). Murphy (1982) found that a lack of a capacity for intimacy lifelong, which is probably a personality trait, was a risk factor for depression in later life. Character and personality traits also interact with life events to modify the risk of depression. Positive coping styles, self-efficacy, and a high level of mastery over the environment are traits which protect the individual from depression (Blazer and Hybels 2005) (see Table 5.1).

In one study, 'cluster C' personality traits (meaning avoidant, dependent, perfectionist, and/or self-defeating in nature) adversely influenced the outcome of depressive disorder in patients aged 60 and above. Compared to patients with non-'cluster C' personality, those with the trait were as likely to respond to treatment but did so more slowly and experienced greater functional impairment (Morse and Robins 2005). This exemplifies the idea of multiple factors, both organic and non-organic, influencing depression and, in this case, pointing towards specific groups of patients who might benefit from a psychological intervention, in addition to an antidepressant. Given the limited availability of psychological therapies, this kind of targeting could be important.

The increased awareness of childhood abuse, including sexual abuse, as a risk factor for depression should not be overlooked just because the patient is older. Strategies which may have enabled coping with adversity earlier in life may break down under ill health, loss, or other threatening life events, resurrecting memories of abuse.

5.1.6 **Psychosocial factors**

Poverty, poor social support, and social isolation are risk factors for depression in later life. A vicious cycle can be engendered, as low socio-economic status and limited access to appropriate treatments tend to go together (Arean and Reynolds 2005). Being a victim of crime is also linked to socio-economic status, making it too a risk factor (Arean and Reynolds 2005). The fear of becoming a victim of crime may be almost as disabling as becoming one, since fear reinforces lifestyles which promote depression, such as isolation and avoidance of outside activity.

5.1.7 **Ethnic and cultural factors**

Acculturation refers to how individuals respond to a dominant culture. This affects the detection of depression, the uptake of mental health services, and the acceptability of treatment. Among older adults, lower levels of acculturation typically lead to a lower likelihood of detecting depression and lower rates of usage of antidepressants. Among ethnic minorities, barriers to the acceptance of mental health care include stigma, concerns about financial re-imbursement (in some health systems), limited local access to specialist mental health services, distrust of mental health providers, and culturally inappropriate services (Unützer et al. 1999).

5.1.8 **Caregiving**

Given the increase in dementia and long-term medical conditions in the population, this deserves emphasis as a risk factor for depression. Ballard *et al.* (1996) reported a quarter of caregivers of those with dementia were depressed and many had persistent symptoms. Factors associated with depression in caregivers include depression in the designated patient and associated problem behaviours. Financial strain adds to the risk (Blazer and Hybels 2005).

5.2 **Precipitating factors**

5.2.1 **Life events**

Table 5.3 lists the more common life events and stressors associated with late-life depressive disorder. In a population of 119 people suffering from depressive disorder,

Table 5.3 Common causes of life events and chronic stress	
Life events	**Chronic stress**
Bereavement Separation Acute physical illness Medical illness or threat to life of someone close Sudden homelessness or having to move into a care home Major financial crisis Negative interactions with family member or friend Loss of 'significant other' (including a pet)	Declining health and mobility Physical dependence Sensory loss, cognitive decline Housing problems Major problems affecting family member Marital difficulties Socio-economic decline Problems at work; retirement Caring for a chronically ill and dependant family member

Murphy (1982) found that 48% had experienced at least one severe life event in the preceding year, compared to 23% of a control group. These were threatening and often involved loss, including bereavement due to the loss of someone close or even a loved pet; life-threatening illness to oneself or someone close; major financial problems; and having to give up one's home suddenly, usually after a serious illness. In addition, major social difficulties (as distinct from sudden events), lasting for 2 years or more, were also significantly associated with depression.

If adversity alone was sufficient to 'explain' depression, then eventually all old people would fall victim to it. Yet, a quarter of Murphy's control group had suffered a major adverse life event and did not develop depression. Not all adverse events are followed by depression; not all depressions are preceded by adverse life events. An uncritical acceptance that a particular life event 'caused' depression can lead to overlooking an undiagnosed medical problem which may be causal (see Table 5.2).

5.2.2 **Bereavement**

Bereavement is a common trigger for depressive disorder in later life. The symptoms of grief and depression often overlap, although grief is dominated by feelings of emptiness and loss which come in waves ('pangs'). The mood in major depression is more persistent and pervasive. In brief, in the first month, low mood, anorexia, insomnia, crying bouts, fatigue, loss of interest, and guilt are common. The latter is typically a rumination about what might have been done to save the person. Suicidal thinking is rare at this stage. After 12 months, somatic symptoms have usually improved, although low mood and poor sleep may persist. The persistence of earlier symptoms is one sign that a bereavement is now complicated by depressive disorder. Other symptoms associated with depression complicating grief include: persistent suicidal thoughts or wishing oneself dead, pervasive guilt (not merely remorse over what more might have been done to prevent death), persistent feelings of worthlessness or hopelessness, 'mummification' (maintaining grief by keeping everything the same), and psychomotor retardation.

A controversial change in DSM-V (American Psychiatric Association 2013) is to remove the so-called 'bereavement exclusion' whereby, in the first 2 months after bereavement, the presence of depressive symptoms are attributed to grief, not major

Table 5.4 Normal grief and major depression

	Normal grief	Major depression
Mood	Sad, tearful, 'emptiness'	Depressed and anhedonic
Thinking	Remorse, fleeting suicidal thoughts—often a wish to 'join' the deceased, rather than commit suicide; preserved self-esteem	Pervasive guilt, persistent suicidal ideation; possibly delusions, feelings of worthlessness
Biological symptoms	Initial insomnia and poor appetite	Persistent insomnia and poor appetite
Function	Temporary problems in function	Persistent and marked impairment in function

depression, unless they are unrelenting, impairing function, or involving psychotic or suicidal thinking. Underlying the removal of the 'bereavement exclusion' is a concern to address the underdiagnosis of major depression. Opponents argue that it medicalizes normal grief. In a footnote in the major depressive disorder section, DSM-V explains that sadness with mild depression, in the face of loss, should not necessarily be viewed a major depression. Clinicians will, therefore, need to exercise a lot of discretion, and Table 5.4 summarizes the main differences between normal grief and major depression.

5.2.3 **Medication**

Many medications (see Table 5.2) are associated with depression, although it is difficult to prove a causal relationship. In a study from Holland, Dhondt *et al.* (2002) examined a large epidemiological database and found that non-selective beta-blockers, calcium channel antihypertensives, systemic steroids, and benzodiazepines were all aetiologically relevant to late-life depression. Self-medication with alcohol may lead to depression or aggravate it. Some reports have suggested that non-steroidal anti-inflammatory drugs (NSAIDs) may interfere with the efficacy of antidepressants. A recent report has not confirmed this (Uher *et al.* 2012).

5.3 **Protective factors**

Relatively little is known about factors which protect against late-life depression (see Table 5.1). If the lack of a confidant leads to depression (Murphy 1982), does the availability of close relationships offer protection from depression? Possibly, but what seems to matter is not merely the availability of such relationships, but whether they are perceived as close and supportive (Blazer and Hybels 2005).

Adaptive coping styles and psychological resilience are further individual factors which may lessen the chances of depression after adversity or stress (Arean and Reynolds 2005). Resilience means the ability to make sense of events, accept one's existence, and carry on with life.

Affiliation and belonging are also important. Religious observance has been shown to protect against depression in older adults in both Western and Eastern cultures (Blazer 2003). Positive events, such as a new grandchild, may protect against depression.

5.4 Neurobiological factors in late-life depression

Although there are multiple pathways to depression, the final changes must occur in the brain. This section covers what is known about the brain in late-life depression.

The biological theory of depression dates back to the 1960s with the amine hypothesis which proposed that brain deficiency of noradrenaline and serotonin (5HT) caused depression. Nowadays, the emphasis is on neurotransmitter systems, rather than single chemicals. These include dopamine pathways, corticotropin-releasing factor (CRF), thyrotropin-releasing hormone (TRH), and growth hormone-releasing factor (GHRF), along with their associated neurohormonal systems, such as the hypothalamic-pituitary-adrenal (HPA) axis. The role of immune and inflammatory responses is also increasingly recognized, since complex interactions occur between the HPA axis and the immune and inflammatory systems.

5.4.1 Biogenic amines

Noradrenaline is associated with attention, memory, concentration, and states of arousal; serotonin with impulse control, sex drive, appetite, and mood; whilst dopamine is concerned with motivation, pleasure-seeking, exploratory behaviour, and reward-mediated behaviour from activities, such as food, sex, and social interaction. Since the ageing brain atrophies, it is reasonable to propose that amine deficiency proceeds with age. This, though, is controversial, as a modern understanding of depression has moved to knowledge of receptor function. For example, autoreceptor binding was dysfunctional in one study of late-life depression and associated with failure to respond to antidepressant medication (Meltzer *et al.* 2004).

5.4.2 Neuroendocrine changes

At all ages, depression is associated with hyperactivity and dysregulation of the HPA axis. Ageing is associated with increasing cortisol levels and cortisol non-suppression. As mentioned earlier, hippocampal atrophy has been linked to chronic depression via cortisol stress. Corticotropin-releasing hormone (CRH) is secreted by the hypothalamus, and it has been shown that CRH mRNA levels in the paraventricular nucleus of elderly depressed patients are higher than the levels in Alzheimer's disease patients (also elevated) and very much higher than normal controls (Raadsheer *et al.* 1995). This has led to speculation that hyperactivation of paraventricular CRH neurons may contribute to the aetiology of late-life depression.

Early life trauma may lead to long-term hypersensitivity of the HPA and CRF systems, which is the basis of the 'stress-diathesis' model of depression. Genetic predisposition, coupled with early stress in critical phases of development, may lead to an individual more vulnerable to developing depression and anxiety upon further exposure to stress. In a study of over 800 singletons born in the 1920s who were interviewed at an average age of 68, Thompson *et al.* (2001) found that the odds ratio for depression among men, but not women, rose incrementally with decreasing birthweight. This could be mediated by faulty programming of the HPA axis very early in life.

5.4.3 Immune and inflammatory changes

Excessive or prolonged exposure to glucocorticoids can compromise the immune system as well as mechanisms of inflammation. In late-life depression, there is evidence of increase in pro-inflammatory markers, but it is not known which came first, the inflammatory changes or the depression (Teper and O'Brien 2007). Inflammatory processes may also mediate the susceptibility of those with late-life depression to cognitive impairment (Viscogliosi *et al.* 2013).

5.4.4 **The vascular depression hypothesis**

For many years, clinicians have suspected that cerebrovascular disease may be relevant to late-life depression. The vascular depression hypothesis proposes that vascular brain disease may predispose to, precipitate, or perpetuate late-life depression (Alexopoulos 2005). Features of vascular depression (compared to non-vascular cases) include less depressive ideation, more psychomotor retardation, poorer insight, executive dysfunction, greater disability, and an onset usually after aged 60. In addition, magnetic resonance imaging (MRI) has shown that patients with late-life depression have a higher rate of hyperintensities in the deep white matter and basal ganglia, compared to control subjects, with the greatest effects seen in late-onset cases. These data have been supplemented by large epidemiological studies which confirm that the severity and location (especially in the basal ganglia) of white matter lesions (WML) are likely to be of causal relevance in late-life depression (Baldwin 2005).

Although there are several causes of WML, a reasonable assumption is that, in depressed patients, they reflect cerebral ischaemia. However, a clear-cut association between the symptoms of vascular depression and common cerebrovascular risk factors (such as hypertension, smoking, hyperlipidaemia, and diabetes) is lacking, as some studies have shown associations and others have not. This does not rule out ischaemia, since chronic hypoperfusion (rather than infarction) may be the causal problem. Brain hypoperfusion is not readily detected by 'bedside' measures of cerebrovascular function, so more sophisticated research will be needed.

In late-life depression, the presence of WML, especially when numerous, severe in extent, or strategically located (as in the basal ganglia), also presages a poorer outcome (Baldwin 2005). WML may also be linked to the syndrome of frailty (wasting, weakness, exhaustion, falls) (Paulson and Lichtenberg 2013). If a significant proportion of late-life depression has a vascular basis, then vasoprotective treatment might possibly help depression. One study showed that, in patients with late-life depression, nimodipine (a drug with vasoprotective properties), when combined with antidepressant medication, led to a reduced time to remission and longer times spent well, compared to a placebo augmentation (Tarangano *et al.* 2005), but this remains to be replicated before such drugs can be recommended.

The vascular depression hypothesis has its critics. Nevertheless, there is strong evidence (to be discussed in Chapter 6) that vascular disease and depression are linked in a bidirectional manner, each increasing the risk of the other. At the very least, the vascular depression hypothesis serves as a reminder that patient management should encompass both psychiatric symptoms and medical co-morbidity, such as vascular disease.

5.4.5 **Neurodegeneration**

Early studies with computerized tomography (CT) showed that brain atrophy occurs in patients with late-life depression. Atrophy and ischaemia may represent alternate pathways to depression (Baldwin 2005).

5.4.6 **Functional imaging and EEG**

The electroencephalogram (EEG) is not a useful investigation in depression unless to help rule out organic brain disease, such as a delirium or dementia. The P300 paradigm uses evoked responses to assess physiological correlates of psychomotor slowing via the EEG. It is an event-related potential recorded via the EEG in the form of a positive deflection in voltage at a latency of roughly 300 ms in the EEG. It may serve as a proxy for superior limbic function, and longer latencies have been found in late-life depression with executive dysfunction. This interesting technology has not yet found an application in clinical practice.

Abnormalities in regional cerebral blood flow (rCBF), using positron emission tomography (PET), in middle-aged and elderly depressed subjects have been reported (Bench *et al.* 1992). Regions particularly affected are the left anterior cingulate gyrus and left dorsolateral pre-frontal cortex. In patients with both depression and cognitive impairment, reduced flow to the left anterior medial pre-frontal gyrus and increased flow to the cerebellar vermis occur. Distinct differences in patterns of blood perfusion in depressed patients, with and without cognitive impairment, help understanding of the cerebral basis of altered cognition in depression.

Single photon emission computerized tomography (SPECT) uses a radioactive tracer, such as 99mTc-hexamethylpropylene amine oxime. There are few studies of older depressed patients, but there is some evidence for a reduction in cerebral perfusion, mainly involving the frontal cortex, with possible recovery after treatment (Navarro *et al.* 2002).

It is now recognized that distributed neuronal networks, and not just single pathways or neurochemicals, are important in depression. Tekin and Cummings (2002) have suggested that superior limbic structures may regulate attention and cognitive aspects of depression (apathy, psychomotor disturbance, impaired attention, and dysexecutive symptoms); a ventral compartment formed of limbic, paralimbic, and subcortical structures may mediate vegetative and somatic aspects (sleep, appetite, endocrine disturbance); and the rostral cingulate area may regulate interactions between these two.

5.4.7 **Post-mortem findings**

The deep white matter hyperintensities of late-life depression, visualized on MRI, have correlates in brain post-mortem tissue where they are revealed to be ischaemic in origin (Teper and O'Brien 2007). Ischaemic white matter lesions tended to be found mainly in the dorsolateral pre-frontal cortex which fits with the PET data discussed previously.

Finally, since there are multiple pathways to depression in later life, Figure 5.1 illustrates how some of these may interact to cause depression. To support the multiple pathway view of late-life depression, Van den Berg *et al.* (2001) studied 132 older depressed patients and found three distinct pathways: an early-onset group associated with a family history of depression, a late-onset group associated with severe life stresses, and a late-onset group associated with vascular risk factors.

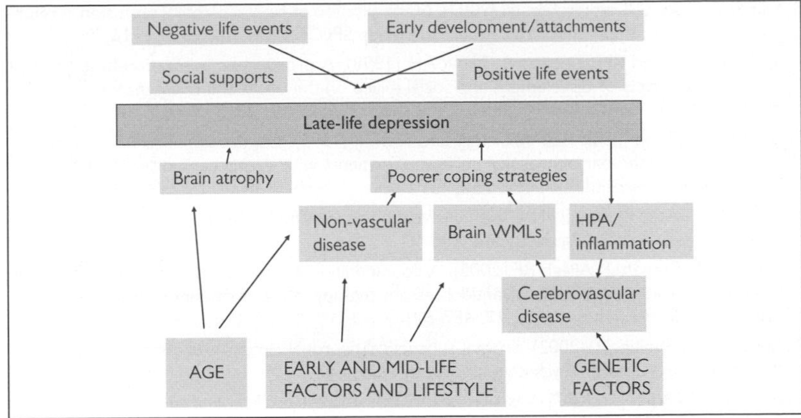

Figure 5.1 Pathways to depression.

Key references

Alexopoulos GS (2005). Depression in the elderly. *The Lancet*, **365**, 1961–70.

American Psychiatric Association (2013). *Diagnostic and statistical manual of mental disorder Fifth edition, DSM V*. American Psychiatric Association, Washington DC.

Arean PA and Reynolds CF (2005). The impact of psychosocial factors on late-life depression. *Biological Psychiatry*, **58**, 277–82.

Baldwin RC (2005). Is vascular depression a distinct sub-type of depressive disorder? A review of causal evidence. *International Journal of Geriatric Psychiatry*, **20**, 1–11.

Ballard CG, Eastwood C, Gahir M, Wilcock G (1996). A follow-up study of depression in the carers of dementia sufferers. *BMJ*, **312**, 947.

Blazer DG (2003). Depression in late life: review and commentary. *Journal of Gerontology: Medical Sciences*, **58A**, 249–65.

Blazer DG and Hybels CF (2005). Origin of depression in later life. *Psychological Medicine*, **35**, 1241–52.

Cole MG and Dendukuri N (2003). Risk factors for elderly community subjects: a systematic review and meta-analysis. *American Journal of Psychiatry*, **160**, 1147–56.

Dhondt TDF, Beekman ATF, Deeg DJH, van Tilburg W (2002). Iatrogenic depression in the elderly. Results from a community-based study in the Netherlands. *Social Psychiatry and Psychiatric Epidemiology*, **37**, 393–8.

Katona CLE and Shankar KK (2004). Depression in old age. *Reviews in Clinical Gerontology*, **14**, 283–306.

Meltzer CC, Price JC, Mathis CA, *et al.* (2004). Serotonin 1A receptor binding and treatment response in late-life depression. *Neuropsychopharmacology*,**29**, 2258–65.

Morse JQ and Robins CJ (2005). Personality-life event congruence effects in late-life depression. *Journal of Affective Disorders*, **84**, 25–31.

Murphy E (1982). Social origins of depression in old age. *British Journal of Psychiatry*, **141**, 135–42.

Navarro V, Gasto C, Lomena F, *et al.* (2002). Normalisation of frontal cerebral perfusion in remitted elderly major depression: a 12 month follow-up SPECT study. *NeuroImage*, **16**, 781–7.

Prince MJ, Harwood RH, Thomas A, Mann AH (1998). A prospective population-based cohort study of the effects of disablement and social milieu on the onset and maintenance of late-life depression. The Gospel Oak Project VII. *Psychological Medicine*, **28**, 337–50.

Raadsheer FC, Joop J, Van Heerikhuize JJ, Lucassen PJ (1995). Corticotropin-releasing hormone mRNA levels in the paraventricular nucleus of patients with Alzheimer's disease and depression. *Archives of General Psychiatry*, **152**, 1372–6.

Rovner BW, Casten RJ, Hegel MT (2007). Preventing depression in age-related macular degeneration. *Archives of General Psychiatry*, **64**, 886–92.

Tarangano FE, Bagnatti P, Allegri RF (2005). A double-blind, randomized clinical trial to assess the augmentation with nimodipine of antidepressant therapy in the treatment of vascular depression. *International Psychogeriatrics*, **17**, 487–98.

Tekin S and Cummings JL (2002). Frontal-subcortical neuronal circuits and clinical neuropsychiatry: an update. *Journal of Psychosomatic Research*, **53**, 647–54.

Teper E and O'Brien JT (2007). Vascular factors and depression. *International Journal of Geriatric Psychiatry*, **23**, 993–1000.

Thompson C, Syddall H, Rodin I, Osmond C, Barker DJP (2001). Birthweight and the risk of depressive disorder in late life. *British Journal of Psychiatry*, **179**, 450–5.

Uher R, Carver S, Power RA, *et al.* (2012). Non-steroidal anti-inflammatory drugs and efficacy of antidepressants in major depressive disorder. *Psychological Medicine*, **42**, 2027–35.

Unützer J, Katon W, Sullivan M, Miranda J (1999). Treating depressed older adults in primary care: narrowing the gap between efficacy and effectiveness. *The Millbank Quarterly*, **77**, 225–56.

van den Berg MD, Oldehinkel AJ, Bouhuys AL, Brilman EI, Beekman ATF, Ormel J (2001). Depression in later life: three etiologically different subgroups. *Journal of Affective Disorders*,**65**, 19–26.

Viscogliossi G, Andreozzi P, Chiriac JM, *et al.* (2013). Depressive symptoms in older people with metabolic syndrome: is there a relationship to inflammation? *International Journal of Geriatric Psychiatry*, **28**, 242–7.

Chapter 6

Medical co-morbidity and depression in later life

Key points
• A number of physical illnesses, common in older people, are associated with high levels of depressive disorder for, and there is effective treatment • The relationship between depression and physical illness is two-way: each influences the presentation of the other. • Recent knowledge about this interaction has grown rapidly for vascular disease and depression, notably with the concept of 'vascular depression'.

Older patients with depression frequently have co-morbid medical conditions or cognitive impairment or both. This chapter considers how these areas interlink in specific conditions that are common in older people: dementia, stroke, cardiac disease, dia betes mellitus, Parkinson's disease, chronic obstructive pulmonary disease (COPD), cancer, and pain. Management will be covered in Chapter 7, Section 7.9.

6.1 Cognitive impairment and depression

Depression is highly prevalent in dementia. It is known that depression can be an early symptom of dementia, but recent epidemiological studies also show that depressive disorder, particularly where chronic or recurrent, is a risk for dementia. For example, in a study involving over 13,000 subjects averaging 81 years and followed over 6 years, Barnes *et al.* (2012) found the risk of developing dementia (both Alzheimer's and vascular dementia) was increased by depression. Those with midlife depression only had a 20% increase in risk of later dementia; those with late-life depression a 70% increase; whilst those who had experienced both midlife and late-life depression had an 80% risk increase. This was for dementia in general, although subjects with both midlife and late-life depression had a threefold risk of developing vascular dementia.

6.2 Stroke and mood disorder

6.2.1 Depression

Depression develops in around 20% of patients within the first year after a stroke, with a peak prevalence at 3 to 6 months, tailing off after 2 or 3 years (Paranthaman and Baldwin 2006). Post-stroke depression has been shown to be a predictor of impaired quality of life and a risk factor for cognitive decline and poorer functional recovery (Evans *et al.* 2005). Making a diagnosis of depression after a stroke can be difficult, especially in patients with aphasia. The 14-item observer-rated stroke aphasic depression questionnaire hospital version (SADQ-H) is one option (Bennett and Lincoln 2006).

Predisposing factors for post-stroke depression include older age, a history of depressive disorder, the size of infarct, female sex, residual disability, and language impairment. Whether depression itself is a risk factor for later cerebrovascular events, such as stroke, is suggested by the preceding discussion (see Section 6.1) about depression and vascular dementia and supported by the systematic review of Pan *et al.* (2011). How depression might predispose to stroke (or vascular dementia) is not fully understood, but depression is known to affect autonomic function and platelet activation.

Difficulty in adjusting to major disability may be sufficient to trigger depression. However, the unusually high rate of depression after stroke and the fact that the relationship between objective severity of stroke and depression is not a consistent one have led to a localization hypothesis. Specifically, it has been suggested that lesion location closer to the anterior pole of the left hemisphere is a risk factor for depression, possibly via disruption of routes connecting the brainstem with the cortex. However, not all agree with the localization hypothesis (Evans *et al.* 2005).

6.2.2 **Post-stroke emotionalism**

Emotional changes, termed emotionalism, following stroke, have been variously described as 'emotionalism', 'pathological affect', 'lability of mood', and 'emotional incontinence'. In emotionalism, crying (or, rarely, laughing) comes with little or no warning and is hard to control so that the subject cries or laughs in social situations where she or he would not normally have done. It affects 20–25% of survivors in the first 6 months after stroke (Paranthaman and Baldwin 2006). Although it declines in frequency and severity over the first year, at 12 months, about 10–15% of survivors remain affected, with some having persistent problems. Depressed mood and emotionalism can occur together, but most people with emotionalism are not depressed. It can occur following a single cortical stroke or bilateral subcortical strokes. There may be a link to serotonergic mechanisms, as lesions have been noted more commonly in the raphae nuclei, an area rich in serotonergic neurons (Paranthaman and Baldwin 2006).

6.3 **Coronary heart disease and vascular disease**

Depressive symptoms occur in about 15–20% soon after a coronary event (Evans *et al.* 2005). At 2 months, of 804 patients with stable coronary heart disease (CHD), 7.1% met criteria for major depression and 5.3% for generalized anxiety disorder (Frasure-Smith *et al.* 2008). These rates are much higher, compared to the general population.

An epidemiological study of older adults from Holland showed that cardiac patients with minor (sub-threshold) depression had a relative risk of subsequent cardiac mortality of 1.6, rising to 3.0 for those with major depression, after adjustment for confounding factors (Penninx *et al.* 2001). Negative effects on cardiac outcome are seen, whether or not subjects are healthy at baseline, and can last for many years, but the maximum impact is generally within the first year after an acute myocardial infarct.

The evidence for depression as an independent risk factor for vascular events has been sufficiently robust for the American Heart Association to recommend screening for depression in cardiac patients. A caution though is that adjustment for baseline factors, especially left ventricular function, substantially attenuates the association of depression and CHD so that 'reverse causality' (those with more severe baseline CHD being more likely to report depression) cannot be ruled out.

6.3.1 **Possible mechanisms**

Biological explanations include autonomic dysfunction, known to be associated with major depression, leading to sympathetic overactivity and/or parasympathetic underactivity, with decreased heart rate variability, downregulated beta-adrenergic receptors, and decreased baroreflex sensitivity, making the diseased heart more susceptible to arrhythmias. Autonomic imbalance is an independent risk factor for early cardiovascular mortality (Carney *et al*. 2007). Platelets may be more activated in depressed patients with heart disease than in depressed patients without. The vascular endothelium produces local vasoactive agents, including nitric oxide, a vasodilator, and the peptide endothelin, a vasoconstrictor. Endothelial dysfunction is thought to precede and predict atheroma, and there is evidence of impairment in adults with depressive disorder. Lifestyle factors in depression include a reduced likelihood of taking medication, such as antihypertensives and antidepressants, inactivity, lack of exercise, smoking, and excessive alcohol intake. These may mediate the relationship between depression and vascular disease (see Figure 6.1). Finally, those with vascular disease may subtly recognize that something is wrong before it becomes clinically apparent, thereby triggering depression.

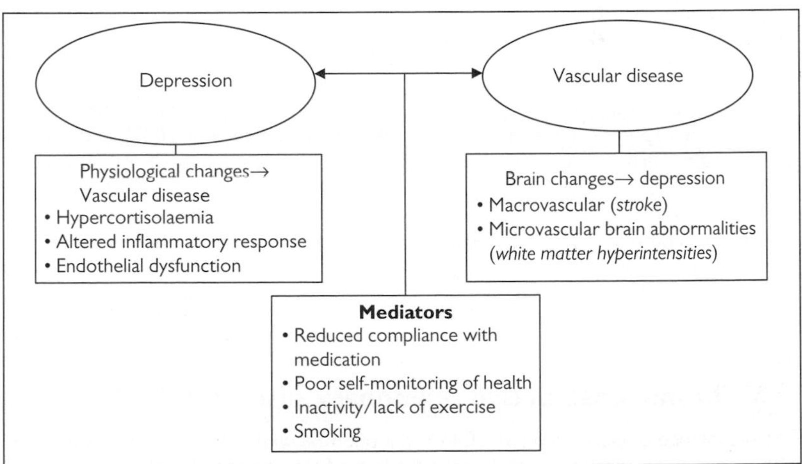

Figure 6.1 Depression and vascular disease.

That depression is bad for arteries is shown by the Pittsburgh Healthy Heart Project (Stewart *et al.* 2007) which indicated that, among 324 adults aged 50–70 years, higher depressive symptoms at baseline were associated with greater 3-year change in carotid intima-media thickness (a measure of atheroma) after adjusting for confounding factors. More recently, Greenstein *et al.* (2010), in a cohort of patients with late-life depression, showed that, compared to controls, those with depression had worse endothelial function, even allowing for baseline vascular risk factors.

6.4 Diabetes

The frequency of type 2 diabetes increases with age. Even after adjustment for diabetes-related co-morbidities, a cohort study of patients aged 70 to 79 years, followed for about 6 years, showed that those with diabetes had a higher level of depression, compared to controls. In this study, HbA1c was a predictor of recurrent depression (Maraldi *et al.* 2007).

There is some evidence of a link between depression and the occurrence of diabetic complications and poorer glycaemic control. Painful neuropathy may be another trigger for depression. Diabetes can cause small vessel pathology in the brain that leads to subcortical encephalopathy, not unlike that seen in vascular depression. This may lead to both cognitive impairment and depressed mood.

6.5 Parkinson's disease

Parkinson's disease causes slowness of movement, rigidity, resting tremor, shuffling gait, and postural instability. Slowness of thought ('bradyphrenia') parallels the physical slowness; the risk of dementia is increased, and significant depressive symptoms occur in about 40% of patients over the course of the illness (Allain *et al.* 2000). Where cognitive impairment is present, depressive symptoms add to its severity. As depression in later life is often associated with cognitive and physical impairment, it is important to take a detailed history to elicit the core symptoms of depression, as described in Chapter 3. Among those with more discrimination in detecting Parkinson's depression are: feelings of guilt, anxiety, anhedonia, and lack of interest plus two somatic symptoms, reduced appetite and early morning wakening (Leentjen *et al.* 2003), and depressive ideation, such as worthlessness, hopelessness, and self-blame (Farabaugh *et al.* 2009). Risk factors for depression in patients with Parkinson's disease include increased physical disability, impaired quality of life, and decreased social interaction. Other factors may be the severity of Parkinson's disease and its duration, although there is an inconsistent relationship between the latter two and depression. Studies have found that depressive symptoms can precede those of motor dysfunction in around 1 in 6 to 1 in 3 patients (Allain *et al.* 2000).

6.6 Chronic obstructive pulmonary disease (COPD)

The prevalence of depression in COPD is about 40%, and, untreated, it is associated with increased physical disability, impaired quality of life, increased health care use, and a higher risk of death.

As with Parkinson's disease, there is considerable overlap with the somatic symptoms of depression. It has been suggested, and to some degree verified by research, that there should be less reliance on somatic symptoms, such as low energy, poor sleep, and weight loss, and more on social withdrawal, fatigue, or loss of energy with brooding or pessimism, and diminished ability to think or concentrate with lack of reactivity to environmental events.

How depression is linked to COPD is unclear. Possible mechanisms include factors related to COPD (level of physical disability and fluctuating mood because of dyspnoea) and behavioural factors (lack of exercise, limited activity, and associated social isolation). Social factors are important, including disruption to social networks caused by repeated hospital admissions (on average, in the UK, moderate-to-severe COPD leads to 3–4 admissions per year) or becoming housebound, either through worsening disability or the need for continuous oxygen treatment.

6.7 Cancer and pain

Both cancer and pain are common in older patients, and depression is a frequent co-morbid condition. Depression can precede a diagnosis of cancer, notably lung and pancreatic cancer, and high rates of depression are seen in breast cancer and head and neck tumours (Evans *et al.* 2005).

Cancer treatment, especially if arduous, and cancer pain are associated with more contact with mental health services (Evans *et al.* 2005), many of which have 'psycho-oncology' specialists. Cytotoxic drugs may trigger depression, and cancer may lead to an increase in pro-inflammatory cytokines which have been linked to depression.

Whether depression increases the risk of cancer is controversial but has been reported in epidemiological research involving older people (Evans *et al.* 2005). One explanation is that depression may work as an immunosuppressant, increasing the chances of a mutation.

Key references

Allain H, Schuck S, Maudit N (2000). Depression in Parkinson's disease. *BMJ*, **320**, 1287–8.

Barnes DE, Yaffe K, Byers AL, McCormick M, Schaefer C, Whitmer RA (2012). Midlife vs late-life depressive symptoms and risk of dementia differential effects for Alzheimer disease and vascular dementia. *Archives of General Psychiatry*, **69**, 493–8.

Bennett HE and Lincoln NB (2006). Potential screening measures for depression and anxiety after stroke. *International Journal of Therapy and Rehabilitation*, **13**, 401–6.

Carney RM, Freedland KE, Stein PK, *et al.* (2007). Heart rate variability and markers of inflammation and coagulation in depressed patients with coronary heart disease. *Journal of Psychosomatic Research*, **62**, 463–7.

Evans DL, Charney DS, Lewis L, *et al.* (2005). Mood disorders in the medically ill: scientific review and recommendations. *Biological Psychiatry*, **58**, 175–89.

Farabaugh AH, Locascio JJ, Yap L, Weintraub D (2009). Pattern of depressive symptoms in Parkinson's disease. *Psychosomatics*, **50**, 448–54.

Frasure-Smith N and Lespérance F (2008). Depression and anxiety as predictors of 2-year cardiac events in patients with stable coronary artery disease. *Archives of General Psychiatry*, **65**, 62–71.

Greenstein A, Paranthaman R, Burns AS, *et al.* (2010). Cerebral microvascular damage in elderly depressed patients is associated with structural and functional abnormalities of subcutaneous small arteries. *Hypertension*, **56**, 734–40.

Leentjens AF, Marinus J, Van Hilten JJ (2003). The contribution of somatic symptoms to the diagnosis of depressive disorder in Parkinson's disease: a discriminant analytic approach. *Journal of Neuropsychiatry and Clinical Neurosciences*, **15**, 74–7.

Maraldi C, Volpato S, Penninx BW, *et al.* (2007). Diabetes mellitus, glycemic control, and incident depressive symptoms among 70- to 79-year-old persons: the health, aging, and body composition study. *Archives of Internal Medicine*, **167**, 1137–44.

Pan A, Sun Q, Okereke OI, Rexrode KM, Hu FB (2011). Depression and risk of stroke morbidity and mortality. *Journal of the American Medical Association*, **306**, 1241–9.

Paranthaman R and Baldwin RC (2006). Treatments of psychiatric syndromes due to cerebrovascular disease. *International Review of Psychiatry*, **18**, 453–70.

Penninx BWJH, Beekman ATF, Honig A, *et al.* (2001). Depression and cardiac mortality results from a community-based longitudinal study. *Archives of General Psychiatry*, **58**, 221–7.

Stage KB, Middleboe T, Stage TB, Sørensen CH, Sørensen CH (2006).Depression in COPD—management and quality of life considerations. *International Journal of Chronic Obstructive Pulmonary Disease*, **1**, 315–20.

Stewart JS, Janicki DL, Muldoon MF, Sutton-Tyrrell K, Kamarck TW (2007). Negative emotions and 3-year progression of subclinical atherosclerosis. *Archives of General Psychiatry*, **64**, 225–33.

Chapter 7

Assessment and management

Key points

- Antidepressant drugs are effective in older patients with depressive episode, with no important differences in individual drug efficacy.
- Antidepressants are effective in depressed patients with a range of physical co-morbid conditions, although tolerability varies.
- Age should not be a barrier to receiving a psychological therapy.
- For chronic depression, combining antidepressant medication with a psychological intervention increases the chance of recovery.
- CBT does not require extensive modification for older people.
- Supportive psychotherapy is not 'doing nothing'.

7.1 Goals of treatment

In England, the underpinning guidance for the management of depression is clinical guideline 90 (National Institute for Health and Clinical Excellence 2009), which is an update of the earlier guideline 23, published in 2004. Contained within this is the 'stepped care' model, meaning that treatment is delivered through a series of steps, ranging from low intensity/non-specialist care to high intensity/specialist input, depending on the severity and complexity of the case. Working in collaboration with the patient and offering treatment choice, wherever possible, underpin effective management.

Antidepressants, psychological interventions, and electroconvulsive treatment (ECT) all work in older patients, just as they do in younger ones. The goals of treatment are to achieve symptomatic remission and to help the patient achieve optimum function, both physically and socially. A framework for achieving this is illustrated in Table 7.1. Remission means that the patient is back to normal, not just improved. Residual symptoms predispose to relapse and chronicity. For patients with more intractable symptoms or whose care is complex, attaining optimum function will require input from health professionals, such as occupational therapy, physiotherapy, specialist nursing (such as community psychiatric nurses), and social workers. This may require referral to specialist psychiatric services. Keeping the patient well after recovery is a further goal and discussed in Chapter 10.

Table 7.1 Framework to achieve symptomatic remission	
Goal	Ways to achieve
Risk reduction—of suicide or harm from self-neglect	• A risk assessment and monitoring of risk • Prompt referral of urgent cases to a specialist
Remission of all depressive symptoms	• Providing appropriate treatment (usually an antidepressant and/or a psychological treatment) • Giving the patient and his/her supporters timely education about depression and its treatment
To help the patient achieve optimal function	• Enable practical support • Ensure access to appropriate agencies that can help
To treat the whole person, including somatic problems	• Treat coexisting physical health problems • Reduce, wherever possible, the effects of handicap caused by factors, such as chronic disease, sensory impairment, and poor mobility • Observe good prescribing practice for older people (see Section 7.3.1)
To prevent relapse and recurrence	• Educate the patient about staying on medication once feeling better • Continuation treatment (staying on treatment after recovery) • Maintenance treatment (preventive treatment) (see Chapter 10)

7.2 **Assessing the patient**

7.2.1 **General assessment**

Assessment starts with the history of symptoms and the mental state examination. It is important to screen for cognitive impairment. This can be undertaken by using the Montreal cognitive assessment 'MoCA' (Nasredinne *et al.* 2005) or the briefer 6-item orientation-memory-concentration (OMC) (Brooke and Bullock 1999) (see also Chapter 8.1). The MoCa can be downloaded from: <http://www.mocatest.org/default.asp>, along with scoring instructions. Provided it is used for clinical purposes, copyright permission is not required.

A physical examination focused on clues from the history should be carried out, for example, neurological examination in patients complaining of cognitive impairment. Laboratory investigation (see Table 7.2) should include haemoglobin and red blood cell counts, which may point to B_{12} deficiency or alcohol misuse. B_{12} and folate estimation should be undertaken in a first episode. Red cell folate gives more information regarding long-term folate stores. Older people can decompensate quite quickly, as they have limited physiological reserve, so that severe depression can lead to under-nutrition or dehydration. These changes occur much more rapidly than in younger patients. An elevated calcium is occasionally associated with depression, as in primary hyperparathyroidism or metastatic cancer, both of which can cause depressed mood, even before the underlying diagnosis is made. Hypothyroidism may be overlooked in the elderly, and 'apathetic hyperthyroidism' can be mistaken for depression. In theory, neurosyphilis can cause depression. This is exceedingly rare nowadays, although the incidence of syphilis is once again on the increase in some countries. There should be

Table 7.2 Investigations for depression in later life		
Investigation	First episode	Recurrence
Full blood count	Yes	Yes
Urea and electrolytes	Yes	Yes
Calcium	Yes	Yes
Thyroid function	Yes	If clinically indicated or more than 12 months elapsed
B_{12}	Yes	If clinically indicated, or more than 12 months elapsed
Folate	Yes	If clinically indicated (for example, recent poor diet)
Liver function	Yes	If indicated (for example, suspected or known alcohol misuse)
Syphilitic serology	If clinically indicated (for example, relevant neurological symptoms)	Only if clinically indicated
CT (brain)	If clinically indicated	If clinically indicated
EEG	If clinically indicated	If clinically indicated

an adequate clinical reason for conducting neurosyphilis testing in a patient presenting with depression, for example, relevant neurological signs, and the clinician should be prepared to discuss this with the patient. The electroencephalogram (EEG) shows no specific changes in depression but can help to differentiate it from dementia or delirium. Neuroimaging in affective disorders is done largely to rule out a space-occupying lesion and in treatment-resistant cases where vascular brain disease is suspected.

7.2.2 **Assessment of executive function**

There are a number of neuropsychological tests or test batteries which can point to executive cognitive problems, which are not uncommon in late-life depression (see Section 3.2). Verbal fluency (letter fluency and category naming) is a sensitive screening test of executive dysfunction in late-life depression (Alexopoulos 2005). Other 'bedside' tests can be carried out if the syndrome is suspected (see Box 7.1). Examine the patient for a grasp reflex by gently scratching the inside of each palm, looking for evidence of grasping. After demonstrating yourself, ask the patient to carry out the action of making a fist, then a cutting motion with the side of the hand, and finally slapping the palm downwards (known as the Luria motor sequencing task). The patient should be able to carry out three sequences in each hand smoothly. Draw a sequence of alternating squares and triangles, using a single line, and ask the patient to do the same; this degrades with frontal executive impairment. The controlled oral word association test is a measure of self-monitoring, verbal fluency, categorization, and initiation. Ask the patient to generate as many words as he or she can think of with three different phonemic letter cues (most often, F, A, and S or C, F, and L), each in a 60-second period. A total raw score of below 30 for patients aged 70 and above with less than 15 years of education suggests impairment. For animal naming, a score below 12 is suspicious

Box 7.1 Brief screening for dysexecutive syndrome

Grasp reflex
Luria hand motor sequencing task
Line drawing:

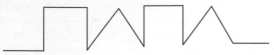

Verbal fluency:

- Controlled oral word association test.
- Animal naming.

(Gladsjo *et al.* 1999). However, educational attainment can affect scores, so they must be treated only as a guide.

Assessing severity is discussed in Section 8.2, with examples in the Appendix.

7.3 **Pharmacotherapy**

7.3.1 **Pharmacological considerations in ageing**

The most important consideration is to recognize that inter-individual difference in drug handling is much greater in older than younger adults (Lotrich and Pollock 2005). Pharmacodynamic considerations include alterations in receptor numbers and affinity and in homeostatic mechanisms. Usually, this leads to increased sensitivity to various side effects at relatively low concentrations of antidepressants. An example is the higher risk of anticholinergic side effects with tricyclic antidepressants (TCAs). Changes in pharmacodynamics may lead to impaired orthostatic responses, impaired thermoregulation, and a risk of delirium. However, altered pharmacodynamics may also be responsible for a decrease in responsiveness to some drugs.

Pharmacokinetic response is affected by reduced renal clearance of the main, and any active, metabolites, diminished microsomal metabolism (involving the P450 systems), a smaller liver mass, reduced hepatic blood flow, and age-related decrements in total albumin and plasma binding. Genetic variation has also been shown to differentially affect the metabolism of antidepressants.

Good prescribing practice for older adults is the best way to put this knowledge into practice. Taylor *et al.* (2012) suggest: avoid drugs which block α_1 adrenoreceptors, have anticholinergic properties, are very sedative, or markedly affect P450 enzyme systems (see Table 7.4); try to minimize the number of drugs given and the number of times per day, and start at low dose first ('start low, go slow'). However, with newer drugs, where the therapeutic dose is close to the starting dose, prolonged dose titration is usually unnecessary.

The management of depressive disorder is divided into three stages (see Chapter 10). Acute treatment refers to the period from initiation of treatment, via improvement, to remission. This usually covers a matter of weeks.

A number of studies indicate that psychotic depression requires treatment with both an antidepressant and an antipsychotic drug, or electroconvulsive therapy (ECT). This will invariably require specialist management.

7.3.2 **Efficacy**

A Cochrane review found that the main classes of antidepressants are all efficacious in late-life depression (Mottram *et al.* 2006) but that serotonin reuptake inhibitors resulted in fewer patients dropping out of treatment, compared to tricyclic drugs, on account of side effects. However, these data are now quite old. A more recent meta-analysis, which included some newer drugs, confirmed this but highlighted a more marginal response for older (over 65) versus younger patients (Tedeschini *et al.* 2011). Furthermore, the goal of remission, important to avoid chronicity, becomes harder to achieve with ageing (Kok *et al.* 2012). This is not to be negative but to emphasize the importance of a logical framework consistently applied for treating older patients (Kok *et al.* 2008) (see Section 7.5).

7.3.3 **Starting treatment**

7.3.3.1 Consent and capacity

It is important to check and record that the patient understands the proposed treatment and agrees to it. Details about mental capacity and its assessment are beyond the scope of this book. In England, the Mental Capacity Act (2005) sets the legal framework. Information is available on the Department of Justice website <http://www.justice.gov.uk/protecting-the-vulnerable/mental-capacity-act>. A summary of key points is listed in Box 7.2. Patients with severe depression or depression with dementia may have to be treated under this legal framework if it is in the person's best interests. Involvement with caregivers and relatives is important, but, unless the patient lacks mental capacity and it is in their best interests, this should always be with the patient's permission.

In England, from April 2009, an amendment to the Mental Capacity Act (2005) means that procedures must be adopted for incapacitous persons whose best interests regarding care and treatment can only be met via interventions in a hospital or registered care home which lead to them being deprived of their liberty. The relevant website is: <http://www.scie.org.uk/publications/ataglance/ataglance43.asp>.

Again, it is possible that some severely depressed patients and some patients with depression complicating dementia or another organic brain syndrome could be affected.

Mental health legislation exists for patients who refuse treatment because of a disordered state of mind (which may include severe depression) and may, as a consequence, suffer harm to themselves, others, or risk a serious deterioration in their health. In England, this is the Mental Health Act 2007 (<http://www.legislation.gov.uk/ukpga/2007/12/contents>).

7.3.3.2 Discussion with the patient

Patients worry that antidepressants are addictive and that depression is 'senility' or an inevitable sign of dementia. Reassurance and encouragement to stick with the treatment are important: the patient must be helped to understand that results take time; otherwise, they will give up early. Goals of treatment should be discussed and agreed with the patient (see Table 7.1). Commonly occurring side effects should be explained.

Box 7.2 Principles and guidance about capacity assessments from Mental Capacity Act (2005) in England

- Assume a person has capacity unless proved otherwise.
- Do not treat people as incapable of making a decision unless you have tried all you can to help them.
- Do not treat someone as incapable of making a decision because their decision may seem unwise.
- Do things or take decisions for people without capacity in their best interests.
- Before doing something to someone or making a decision on their behalf, consider whether you could achieve the outcome in a less restrictive way.
- Be clear about the decision to be made and who is the decision maker.
- The key principle is that all decisions must be made in the best interests of the person who lacks capacity, taking into consideration all relevant circumstances.
- The Act does not define best interests but does give a checklist:
  - Must involve the person who lacks capacity.
  - Have regard for past and present wishes and feelings.
  - Consult with others who are involved in the care of the person.
  - Undertake the assessment under circumstances which maximize the person's capabilities.
  - Document the decision, and review it, as necessary.

Box 7.3 Practical aspects of concordance in treatment

- Understanding the patient's and caregiver's perception of what depression is.
- Explaining what depression is and what it is not (for example, 'weakness of character').
- Clarifying attribution of symptoms (for example, 'it's all down to my heart, doctor').
- Explaining side effects.
- Explaining delay in onset.
- Agreeing management plan and treatment goals.
- Involving family/supporters with consent of the patient.

There is a high placebo response rate to antidepressants. This is probably because placebo treatment involves much more than a pill. In clinical trials, to establish the efficacy of a compound, participants will see members of the research team regularly, and they will provide empathic listening and informal support. These 'non-specific' factors in the treatment of late-life depressive disorder are nowadays widely recognized as key components of care. Likely ingredients include: having a plausible treatment delivered by someone perceived as an expert who is enthusiastic about it and who takes depression seriously; the expectation of improvement; the positive regard of the prescriber towards the patient; listening with empathy; encouraging verbalization of distress; and, perhaps especially important in older adults, encouragement to undertake purposeful activity to counter apathy and withdrawal.

Building the therapeutic relationship in this way is important in establishing treatment concordance. Not taking medication is the major cause of treatment failure. Box 7.3 lists key aspects of concordance to consider.

7.4 **Pharmacological management in the acute phase**

7.4.1 **Classification of antidepressants used to treat older adults**

A classification of antidepressants is shown in Box 7.4.

7.4.2 **Individual drugs and dosages**

The main mode of action of antidepressants and the average starting and therapeutic dosages are listed in Table 7.3. With so many antidepressants to choose from, the principle is to match the antidepressant to the patient, taking into account tolerability, safety, likely side effects, drug interactions, and contraindications. The three most

Box 7.4 Classification of antidepressants

Older tricyclics
Secondary amines (nortriptyline, desipramine)
Tertiary amines (imipramine, amitriptyline, dosulepin, clomipramine)

Newer tricyclics
Lofepramine

Atypical antidepressants
Trazodone, mianserin

Monoamine oxidase inhibitors (non-reversible)
Phenelzine
Tranylcypramine

Reversible inhibitors of monoamine oxidase A ('RIMA' agents)
Moclobemide

Selective serotonin reuptake inhibitors (SSRIs)
Fluvoxamine, fluoxetine, paroxetine, sertraline, citalopram, escitalopram

Noradrenaline and specific serotonin antidepressants (NASSa)
Mirtazapine

Noradrenaline reuptake inihibitors (NARI)*
Reboxetine

Aminoketone
Bupropion

Serotonin/noradrenaline reuptake inhibitors (SNRI)
Venlafaxine
Duloxetine

Melatonergic
Agomelatine

*Not recommended for older adults in the UK because of lack of evidence at the time of granting a licence.

Table 7.3 Mode of action, side effect profiles, and dosages of the main antidepressants used to treat late-life depression in the UK (see also Baldwin et al. 2002; Unützer 2007)

Drug	Main mode of action	Main side effects	Starting dosage (mg)	Average daily dose (mg)
Amitriptyline	NA++ 5HT+	Sedation Anticholinergic, postural hypotension, tachycardia/arrhythmia	25–50	75–100*
Imipramine	NA++ 5HT+	As for amitriptyline but less sedation	25	75–100*
Nortriptyline	NA++ 5HT+	As for amitriptyline but less sedation, anticholinergic effects and hypotension	10 tds	75–100*
Dosulepin	NA++ 5HT+	As for amitriptyline	50–75	75–150*
Lofepramine	NA++ 5HT+	As for amitriptyline but less sedation, anticholinergic effects, hypotension, and cardiac problems	70–140	70–210
Trazodone	$5HT_2$	Sedation, dizziness, headache	100	300–400
Citalopram	5HT	Nausea, vomiting, dyspepsia, abdominal pain, diarrhoea, headache, sexual dysfunction; risk of gastric bleeding; inappropriate ADH secretion	20	20
Sertraline	5HT	As for citalopram	50	100–200
Fluoxetine	5HT	As for citalopram but insomnia and agitation more common	20	20*
Paroxetine	5HT	As for citalopram but sedation and anticholinergic effects may occur	20	20
Fluvoxamine	5HT	As for citalopram but nausea more common	50–100	100–200
Escitalopram	5HT	As for citalopram	5	10
Moclobemide	MAO	Sleep disturbance, nausea, agitation	300	300–400
Venlafaxine	NA 5HT	Nausea, insomnia, dizziness, dry mouth, somnolence, hyper- and hypotension	75	150**
Duloxetine	NA 5HT	Nausea, insomnia, dizziness	30	60–90
Mirtazapine	α_2 blocking selective antagonist of $5HT_2$ and $5HT_3$ receptors	Increased appetite, weight gain, somnolence, headache	15	30–45

Table 7.3 (Continued)				
Drug	Main mode of action	Main side effects	Starting dosage (mg)	Average daily dose (mg)
Bupropion	Noradrenaline/dopamine reuptake inhibition	Seizures, hypertension; not sedative and less likely to cause weight gain or sexual side effects	150 bd (as extended release)	300
Agomelatine	Melatonergic agonist (MT 1 and 2 receptors); $5HT_{2c}$ antagonist	Dizziness, sickness, somnolence	25	25–50

NA, noradrenaline; 5HT, serotonin, MAO, monoamine oxidase inhibitor.

* These are average doses. Some patients will require higher dosages, depending on response and tolerability.

** Titration up to higher dosages is common in specialist care.

+ indicates relative strength of monoamine effect.

Table 7.4 Inhibition of P450 enzymes by SSRIs (see also Taylor et al. 2012)				
Enzyme group inhibited by SSRI	IA2	2C9	2D6	3A
Example of substrate	Caffeine	Phenytoin	Tricyclics	Benzodiazepines
Fluoxetine	+	++	+++	++
Sertraline	+	+	+	+
Paroxetine	+	+	+++	+
Citalopram	+	0	+	0
Escitalopram	0	0	0	0
Fluvoxamine	+++	++	+	++

Degree of inhibition: 0, minimal; +, mild inhibition; ++, moderate inhibition; +++, strong inhibition.

commonly prescribed SSRIs citalopram, sertraline, and escitalopram are non-sedative, whereas mirtazapine is sedative and may be helpful for depression-associated insomnia. Note that bupropion is only licensed in the US for the treatment of depression. It is licensed in the UK only for the treatment of smoking cessation.

7.4.3 Side effects and interactions

The P450 enzyme systems are the main mode of metabolism. Via the 2D6 system, prescription of SSRIs, such as paroxetine and fluoxetine, and the dual-acting drug duloxetine can lead to inhibition of the metabolism of tricyclic antidepressants, antipsychotics, lipophilic beta-blockers, some analgesics (such as codeine), some anti-arrhythmics, and triazolobenzodiazepines, such as alprazolam. Adverse interactions between SSRIs and TCAs occur because each may inhibit the metabolism of the other. Via the 2C and 3A enzyme systems, fluoxetine and paroxetine can inhibit the metabolism of benzodiazepines, calcium channel blockers, cisapride, terfenadine, and theophylline and enhance the effects of phenytoin. Table 7.4 shows that citalopram, escitalopram, and sertraline are least likely of the SSRIs to be involved in P450 interactions and are, therefore, often recommended as first-line antidepressants in late-life depression. Venlafaxine acts like an SSRI, with minimal effects on the 2D6 enzyme. Mirtazapine too has minimal effects on 1A2, C9, and 2D6.

Table 7.3 shows the main side effects of antidepressants used to treat late-life depression. Anticholinergic side effects include dry mouth, blurred vision, constipation, and urinary retention and are common with TCA treatment. Cardiotoxicity is a further concern, and it is recommended that an electrocardiogram (ECG) be carried out prior to commencing an older TCA. Cardiac arrhythmia in TCA overdose can be fatal. In medically unwell patients, delirium can occur. Guidance issued by the UK Medicines and Health products Regulatory Authority (MHRA) in 2011 requires that the maximum dosages of citalopram and escitalopram for older patients are 20 and 10 mg, respectively. This is because of evidence that they increase the ECG corrected QT interval (QTc), raising the risk of arrhythmia. Citalopram and escitalopram should not be combined with antipsychotic drugs, most of which can also prolong the QTc interval. Postural hypotension due to adrenergic blockade is a serious problem with TCAs and dual-acting drugs (SNRIs). With the TCAs and mirtazapine, histaminic effects can cause sedation and weight gain. Lofepramine is a second-generation TCA less likely to cause these adverse effects.

With the proviso of keeping to the revised dosages of citalopram and escitalopram, SSRIs are safer than TCAs, but they have their own side effects, including nausea (around 15%), diarrhoea (around 10%), insomnia (5–15%), anxiety and/or agitation (2–15%), headache, weight loss, and sexual dysfunction (an area hardly ever inquired of with older people, hence its prevalence is almost certainly underestimated). SSRIs have minimal impact on cognitive function in older patients with depression and may have less impairment on driving skills than older drugs. Because SSRIs are associated with bleeding risk, gastroprotective medication is recommended for older patients on non-steroidal anti-inflammatory drugs or aspirin or a prior history of ulcer or bleeding problems (see Box 7.5). There are also concerns that SSRIs may reduce bone density through their effects on serotonin transporter in bone tissue (Haney and Warden 2009). To what extent this is clinically relevant is not yet clear, although there are reports of increased falls and hip fracture in patients taking SSRIs (Richards *et al.* 2007) (although depression itself is associated with an increased risk of falls (Mc Veigh *et al.* 2013)). Finally, SSRI drugs can cause restlessness and a temporary increase in suicidal feelings. This is particularly so for young patients, but some older patients experience this too, so they need to be warned about it in the initiation stage of treatment.

Discontinuation symptoms may occur if the antidepressant is stopped suddenly. This is more likely after 4 weeks of treatment and with short half-life drugs. Therefore, it is least likely with fluoxetine and more so with paroxetine and venlafaxine. SSRIs may

Box 7.5 Unwanted effects of antidepressants to be particularly watchful for in older patients

- Delirium
- Postural hypotension
- Gastric bleeding
- Inappropriate ADH secretion
- Falls and/or unsteadiness

cause inappropriate antidiuretic hormone (IADH) secretion, and increased age, female gender, and drugs that lower sodium levels are all risk factors. Symptoms of IADH, which include lethargy, fatigue, and sleep disturbance as well as muscle cramps and headaches, overlap with those of depression.

Moclobemide is tolerated well by older people, and, although a special diet is not required (as with older monoamine oxidase inhibitors), patients should be aware of the drug interactions with painkillers and other antidepressants. Co-prescriptions of moclobemide with tricyclics or SSRIs should be avoided. A washout period of around 4–5 half-lives of the drug and any active metabolite is advised when transferring from a tricyclic or an SSRI to moclobemide (but is not necessary from moclobemide to a tricyclic or an SSRI).

Venlafaxine is generally well tolerated, provided the dose is increased incrementally. Hypertension is a known problem with venlafaxine, but, in older patients, postural hypotension can also occur (see Table 7.3). Venlafaxine is not recommended for patients with heart disease likely to predispose to arrhythmia. Duloxetine, a newer dual-acting antidepressant, has not been shown to be cardiotoxic.

Of other drugs, mirtazapine and trazodone have side effects similar to TCAs. There are occasional reports of priapism with trazodone. Rarely, mirtazapine can cause agranulocytosis, and patients should be told to report symptoms suggestive of this, such as a persistent sore throat or fever.

Agomelatine may cause less sexual side effects and may improve sleep, but it has been shown to be hepatotoxic and requires regular monitoring of liver function.

7.5 Next pharmacological steps for patients not responsive to initial treatment

In a meta-analysis of randomized controlled trials of newer antidepressants involving older adults, the mean response rate was 44% (Nelson *et al.* 2008). Therefore, a high percentage of patients will not respond to their first antidepressant. Box 7.6 shows a strategy to follow before the patient is considered 'resistant' to treatment. The study of Nelson *et al.* (2008) also showed that trials of antidepressants lasting 10–12 weeks

Box 7.6 Strategy for non-responsive patients

(1) If little or no response (<25% reduction in symptoms) by 4 weeks:
   Increase the dose
OR
   If dosage optimal, change to another antidepressant (switch class)
(2) If partial response by 4 weeks:
   Optimize dose (if not already done)
   Continue and review 2–4 weekly
(3) If little further improvement by 8 weeks:
   Consider augmentation (either with medication or a psychological intervention)
OR
   Consider combining antidepressants
(4) At all stages, consider electroconvulsive therapy, if indicated by severity or risks

Box 7.7 A systematic approach to resistant depression

- Review the diagnosis (for example, could this be psychotic depression?).
- Review treatment adequacy (duration, dose, compliance).
- Ensure a logical framework has been used (rational sequential treatment) within a framework or protocol).
- Measure outcome appropriately (for example, symptoms of depression and social recovery from depression may follow different trajectories).
- Address medical co-morbidity (note in late-onset cases, consider vascular depression).
- Address psychiatric morbidity (for example, residual anxiety, insomnia).
- Consider factors in the treatment setting, including family and relationship factors that have been overlooked (for example, avoidance behaviour and over-dependency).

resulted in increased efficacy, compared to those of 6 weeks (the median length for most antidepressant trials). This suggests that older patients take longer to recover. Therefore, one strategy is to increase the length of treatment with the existing antidepressant, as the response rate will go on rising, provided that there has already been a meaningful response.

Box 7.7 shows what to look for before concluding that the patient is 'resistant' to treatment.

7.6 Pharmacological management of resistant depression

There is no universally agreed guideline as to what constitutes resistance to treatment. If there is genuine non-response after two trials of different antidepressants, each of at least 4 weeks' duration at optimum doses, then there are a number of strategies (see Table 7.5) to consider. Persistence pays. In a clinical series, Kok *et al.* (2009), using a rational sequential protocol, showed that sequential regimes of antidepressant therapy eventually produced improvement (over 90%) or recovery (80%) in their patients who had not responded to either venlafaxine or nortriptyline. Many of the strategies require specialist input.

7.6.1 Combining antidepressants

Dodd *et al.* (2005) conducted a literature review (not specific to older patients) on combining antidepressants and suggested that combination treatment helps about 50% of patients not responsive to antidepressant monotherapy. Although generally safe, some adverse reactions were reported, including one report of the serotonergic syndrome (see Box 7.8). For older patients, there are little specific data, and we are reliant on extrapolating from this broader research, always remembering that older patients are more susceptible to adverse effects and drug interactions. Popular combinations include an SSRI plus mirtazapine and venlafaxine plus mirtazapine, but these should only be undertaken by specialists.

Table 7.5 Strategies for resistant depression

Strategy	Example
Optimization (maximize dose/serum level/time)	• Dose increase • Prolong course • Measure/adjust drug concentration (tricyclics only)
Substitution (substitute one antidepressant for another)	• SSRI to SSRI • SSRI to a different class
Augmentation (use of a non-primary antidepressant)	• Lithium • Atypical antipsychotic • Psychological intervention • Tri-iodothyronine (T3)
Combination (use two primary antidepressants together)	• SSRI + mirtazapine • Mirtazapine + venlafaxine

Box 7.8 Serotonin syndrome

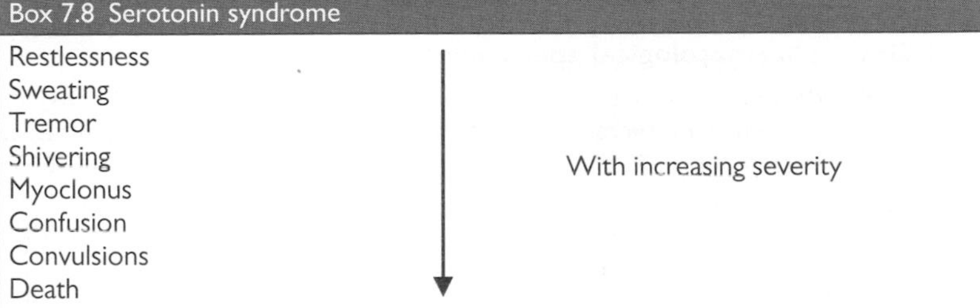

Restlessness
Sweating
Tremor
Shivering
Myoclonus
Confusion
Convulsions
Death
With increasing severity

7.6.2 **Augmentation**

Augmentation refers to adding a drug which is not an antidepressant. Although its use has waned in recent years, lithium augmentation remains an effective treatment for the management of resistant depression. Its use can be difficult in older patients, as side effects and the risk of toxicity are higher. Side effects affecting a quarter or more of older adults on lithium are: polydipsia, polyuria, mild tremor, dry mouth, nausea, and memory impairment. Toxicity (marked tremor, unsteadiness, incoordination, confusion, and altered level of consciousness) may affect 10% of older patients at some point during lithium treatment. The risk is increased by dehydration, such as caused by a chest infection, other febrile illness, or diarrhoea and vomiting. Renal disease is another risk factor, as is treatment with diuretics, non-steroidal anti-inflammatory drugs (NSAIDs), and ACE inhibitors. Do not forget that lithium toxicity has been reported in patients with brain damage, even at serum levels in the therapeutic range; the clinical picture is the best guide. Occasionally, asymptomatic hypercalcaemia and hyperparathyroidism occur, a risk which is highest in those aged over 60 (Lehmann and Lee 2013).

Some geriatric psychiatrists suggest using low-dosage lithium, aiming for a serum level of around 0.35–0.5 mmol/L, instead of the current recommended one of 0.6–0.8 mmol/L for bipolar patients (NICE 2006). It is unclear whether low dosaging is as effective as conventional dosaging. In the study of Kok *et al.* (2009), 22 patients received lithium, with a remission rate of two-thirds, higher than some other recent studies of lithium augmentation, but the mean lithium level was 0.82 mmol/L, i.e. in the conventional range.

Although there are limited data specific to older patients, there is growing evidence that augmentation of antidepressants with atypical antipsychotic medication improves outcomes (Nelson and Papakostas 2009)—although there are concerns about longer-term outcomes, especially the metabolic syndrome (altered glycaemic control, dyslipidaemia, obesity, and hypertension) (Jin *et al.* 2013). Therefore, if used, this should generally be under specialist guidance and for short-term treatment only, for example, 4–6 months.

The main role for anticonvulsants in depression is lamotrigine for bipolar depression. Pregabalin, licensed for generalized anxiety disorder, has been shown to be effective in older adults (Montgomery *et al.* 2008). Since residual anxiety is a common intractable problem in treating older adults, the use of this drug adjunctively may have a place in resistant depression. There is some evidence to support this (Karaiskos *et al.* 2013).

7.6.3 **Other pharmacological approaches**

Because of dietary restrictions, traditional monoamine oxidase inhibitors (MAOIs) are rarely used, although there were some early reports of success. Recent interest in transdermal selegiline for depression may revive interest (Goldberg and Thase 2013). Trials are sparse so far, and problematic interactions, much like those of the older MAOIs, can occur at all but the lowest, dose. Moclobemide is different—it is a reversible and selective inhibitor of MAO-A.

L-tryptophan may have a role as an adjunctive therapy in treatment-resistant depression but has been associated with the eosinophilic-myalgic syndrome and a risk of the serotonin syndrome when combined with other antidepressants, such as SSRIs (see Box 7.8).

Thyroid supplementation has been advocated for resistant depression, but there are no data for later-life patients for whom caution would be necessary.

One might think that cholinesterase inhibitors, such as are licensed to treat Alzheimer's disease, could improve cognition in depressed patient, many of whom have some impaired cognition, but there is no evidence to support this (McDermott and Gray 2012).

One of the most interesting developments has been the role of ketamine in improving depressive symptoms. A number of trials are underway, and the early evidence suggests an almost immediate response in resistant depression, but the effects are short-lived.

7.7 **Non-pharmacological strategies**

7.7.1 **Electroconvulsive therapy (ECT)**

Similar to lithium, the use of ECT has declined but less so for older adults, perhaps because it is effective and often better tolerated than multiple medications. Opinion is that bilateral treatment is more effective but associated with a higher risk of memory impairment, the main adverse effect. A common strategy is to start with bilateral placement but switch to unilateral if memory effects become prominent.

Headache and memory loss are the most commonly reported side effects. The latter causes amnesia, particularly around the time of the administration of ECT.

An important drawback with ECT is the high subsequent relapse rate. Evidence suggests giving an antidepressant plus lithium to prevent relapse, and probably the new-generation antipsychotics may help to reduce short-term relapse. Maintenance ECT, often given fortnightly or monthly, can be offered in high-risk groups.

7.7.2 **Repetitive transcranial magnetic stimulation**

Repetitive transcranial magnetic stimulation (rTMS) is a reasonably effective treatment for moderate depressive episode, but high-quality randomized controlled trials (RCTs) in later-life patients are lacking. Frontal atrophy, as can occur in late-life vascular depression, may reduce the response to rTMS in older patients. Jorge *et al.* (2008) studied rTMS in 92 patients with major depression aged over 50, with vascular depression randomized to rTMS (12,000 pulses), rTMS (18,000 pulses), or sham rTMS, over a 10-day period. Using the 18k paradigm, there was a significantly better response in the actively treated group, although remission rates were fairly low in all three groups. Age predicted a poorer response.

7.7.3 **Other strategies**

Psychological interventions (discussed in Section 7.8) should be considered as valid strategies for the augmentation of antidepressants.

Do not forget that exercise is an antidepressant and can help with the highly damaging inertia that afflicts older depressed patients who have not responded quickly to treatment.

Lastly, psychosurgery is still used in a few designated centres. Success is reported, although the patients referred to these centres are usually middle-aged, rather than elderly.

7.8 **Psychological interventions**

Age is no barrier to psychological interventions for depression; for moderate depressive disorder, they are as effective as medication (Pinquart *et al.* 2006). Currently, there is evidence for the efficacy of cognitive behavioural therapy (CBT) and behaviour therapy, interpersonal therapy (IPT), and dynamic psychotherapy. Most research though has been conducted using CBT and IPT. CBT helps the patient in the here and now to understand the links between low mood and both negative cognitions and behaviour. In IPT, the emphasis is on current problems within the interpersonal context. An understanding of past relationships may help but is not a major emphasis. IPT aims to help patients change, rather than to simply understand and accept their current life situation. Mindfulness treatment, based on meditative principles and Buddhism, has been endorsed by the National Institute of Health and Care Excellence in England for the treatment of chronic depression.

Problem-solving treatment (PST) is of proven efficacy in younger patients with mild-to-moderate depression. PST also deals with the here and now, focusing on current difficulties and setting future goals. It is designed to help the patient gain a sense of mastery over difficulties. Behavioural activation is similar to PST and involves scheduling

Box 7.9 Example of simple tools to use for behavioural activation

	Monday	Tuesday	Wednesday	Thursday	Friday	Saturday	Sunday
9–10							
10–11							
11–12							
12–1							
1–2							
2–3							
3–4							
4–5							
5–6							
6–7							
7–8							
8–9							

On this chart, write the activities you aim to do in the next week. Write them on the day and time that you aim to do them. To begin with, write down 1–2 things a day.

On completing each activity, score your feeling of achievement and pleasure, using the following scales:

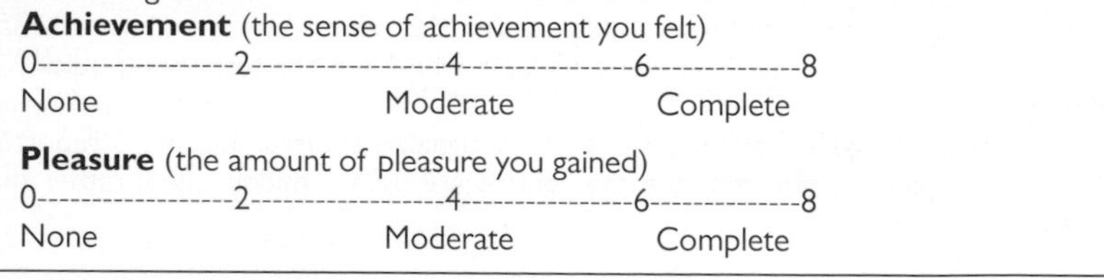

Achievement (the sense of achievement you felt)

0------------------2------------------4----------------6--------------8

None Moderate Complete

Pleasure (the amount of pleasure you gained)

0------------------2------------------4----------------6--------------8

None Moderate Complete

activity on a regular basis and self-evaluating progress. It can help to address the anergia and apathy that sometimes accompany late-life depression. An example of a simple tool which can be used for behavioural activation is shown in Box 7.9.

Of studies which have compared antidepressants drugs with a psychological intervention or with a combination of medication plus a psychological treatment, the combination appears to be more effective than either given alone, and this effect appears stronger in patients with more severe depression. Importantly, this appears to be so in older patients, even where there is a clear trigger, such as bereavement (Reynolds *et al.* 1999).

It is sometimes necessary to modify techniques, such as CBT, with older adults, but the modifications required are not as extensive as is sometimes supposed—older adults adapt well to this approach. Common sense changes include use of repetition, writing things down, and shorter sessions.

Family therapy has been adapted for use with older clients, and there are case reports of its efficacy in both dementia and depression. In an RCT, a family intervention delivered to carers of patients with dementia resulted in significant reduction of

Table 7.6 Strategies for resistant depression

	Depression (NICE CG 90 and 91, 2009) *Treatment phase*	Depression (NICE CG 90 and 91, 2009) *Continuation and relapse prevention*	Bipolar disorder (NICE CG 38, 2006; under review)
Therapeutic interventions	• Group CBT 6–8 weeks), or • Individual CBT (16–20 sessions) • Behavioural activation (16–20 sessions)	• Individual CBT • Mindfulness: group up to 12 months • Psychodynamic therapy (16–20 sessions over 4–6 months)	• If depressed—as for depression • Individual structured: 16 sessions over 6–9 months (entering recovery) • Sleep therapy

stress, burden, and depressive symptoms, with a number-needed-to treat of just two. (Marriott *et al.* 2000).

The utilization of psychological interventions within the National Institute for Health and Care Excellence (NICE) guidelines (England) for depression, depression with a physical illness, and depression occurring in bipolar disorder (guidelines 90, 91, and 38) are shown in Table 7.6. Note that most interventions can be delivered in groups, making for increased efficiency.

Psychological interventions also have a place in relapse prevention. Reynolds *et al.* (1999) found that monthly IPT, given in the continuation phase of treatment, was more effective than routine care, and the combination of IPT with maintenance antidepressant therapy was the most effective of all. However, the same researchers were unable to replicate this in a later study with a group of patients, on average, 10 years older (Reynolds *et al.* 2006). Probably, this was due to cognitive impairment which may, therefore, restrict the efficacy of some psychological approaches in later-life depression.

Last, recent data show that, contrary to what is usually taught, simple forms of psychological therapy (so-called 'low intensity') work as effectively in more severe depression as in less severe depression (Bower *et al.* 2013).

7.9 **Treatment in co-morbidity**

Many of the conditions of later life, both physical and dementia, are associated with a high rate of depression, as discussed in Chapter 6. General guidance for the treatment of depression arising in chronic physical disorder is provided by the NICE guideline 91 (NICE 2009).

7.9.1 **Depression in dementia**

The principles of treating depression associated with dementia are no different from those of 'uncomplicated' depression. However, recent evidence concerning the efficacy of both medication and psychosocial interventions is disappointing. Banerjee *et al.* (2011), in the largest RCT of its kind, showed that neither sertraline nor mirtazapine were more effective than placebo for treating depression associated with Alzheimer's disease. In a cost-benefit analysis (Romeo *et al.* 2013) there was an advantage for mirtazapine, probably because patients slept better on mirtazapine and the carers were, therefore, more likely to sleep and fulfill their daytime tasks. In another study (Munro *et al.* 2012), sertraline had no effect on cognition in patients with depression associated with dementia.

In a further study (Waldorff *et al.* 2012), a semi-tailored intervention with counselling, education, and support for patients with mild Alzheimer's disease and their caregivers did not show any significant effect over usual care after 12 months. Hence, at the present time, we do not have any truly effective interventions for depression in dementia. More positively though, as described in the preceding section, there are effective interventions to relieve the depression of the caregivers.

7.9.2 **Stroke**

A recent review of the literature found only ten randomized controlled trials of antidepressants (fluoxetine, citalopram, sertraline, nortriptyline) in post-stroke depression. There was evidence of efficacy, but the quality and size of the trials were variable (Paranthaman and Baldwin 2006). Stimulants, such as methylphenidate 5 to 10 mg daily, may benefit stroke-related apathy but are not recommended for routine use.

There is little evidence for the efficacy of psychological interventions in post-stroke depression, but this is largely because such studies are difficult to conduct. However, there is emerging evidence that both medication with SSRIs and problem-solving treatment can prevent post-stroke depression (Robinson *et al.* 2008). This can be considered for patients who have a high risk of post-stroke depression, for example, those with a previous history of depression.

Both tricyclic antidepressants and SSRIs are effective in treating emotionalism. There are also reports of the successful use of mirtazapine and venlafaxine. SSRIs are nowadays the recommended first-line treatment on grounds of reduced side effects (Paranthaman and Baldwin 2006). Unlike depression, a response is often seen within the first week, irrespective of lesion location or time since the stroke.

7.9.3 **Coronary heart disease (CHD)**

Treatment of depression with an antidepressant or a psychological intervention produces modest improvements in depression. Because SSRIs decrease platelet function, there is a theoretical reason for thinking that SSRI treatment may reduce cardiac mortality, but no antidepressant treatment trial has demonstrated this.

Tricyclic antidepressants (TCAs) are type 1A anti-arrhythmics, and they can reduce heart rate variability, a factor linked to increased mortality. In Section 7.4.3, mention was made of important guidance regarding cautions with citalopram, escitalopram, or the combination of these drugs with any of the antipsychotics because of the effects on cardiac repolarization. Venlafaxine can increase blood pressure, although, in older patients, it can cause postural hypotension. It should not be used in patients with a significant risk of ventricular arrhythmia. Lithium treatment can potentiate arrhythmia and has been linked to heart block. Currently, the most widely studied antidepressant in cardiac disease, other than the tricyclics, is sertraline, and there is no evidence that it adversely affects cardiac physiology (Castro *et al.* 2013). Bupropion, used in some countries to augment antidepressants, has been shown to reduce the QTc interval (Castro *et al.* 2013).

7.9.4 **Diabetes**

Depression in diabetes is usually treated with an SSRI. TCAs are more likely to impair diabetic control than SSRIs, although fluoxetine should be used with caution as it can cause hypoglycaemia. TCAs can help painful neuropathy. Mirtazapine may cause weight gain (a risk factor for diabetes); lithium toxicity is increased if there is nephropathy, and valproate may give a false positive result on urine testing for glucose. There is also interest in the use of alternative and complementary medicine to improve glycaemic control and mood in diabetic patients. These include Ayurvedic medicine, exercise, mindfulness, yoga, and acupuncture. There is also some evidence of benefits from cognitive behavioural therapy (CBT). However, as with the treatment of depression in heart disease, it has yet to be demonstrated that interventions are disease-modifying (as measured by glycosylated haemoglobin levels).

7.9.5 **Parkinson's disease**

L-dopa has not been shown to improve mood in Parkinson's disease patients. RCT evidence exists for the efficacy of several antidepressants (venlafaxine and paroxetine, Richard *et al.* 2012; nortriptyline, Menza *et al.* 2009). Concerns have been expressed that SSRIs can cause emergent extrapyramidal effects, but this is controversial and not supported by these recent RCTs. The combination of an SSRI and selegiline can lead to the serotonin syndrome (see Box 7.8).

Tianeptine (which increases the presynaptic recapture of 5-hydroxy indoleacetic acid) and moclobemide (a reversible and selective inhibitor of monoamine oxidase) have been used to treat depression in Parkinson's disease, but the evidence is largely empirical. Deep brain stimulation is a treatment for both Parkinson's disease and severe depression, although, paradoxically, it may provoke depression in Parkinson's patients.

Electroconvulsive therapy (ECT) is effective in treating severe depression with Parkinson's disease as well as improving motor symptoms, albeit temporarily. There are some studies of rTMS in depression associated with Parkinson's disease, and further evidence is awaited.

7.9.6 **Chronic obstructive pulmonary disease (COPD)**

There are no high-quality trials of antidepressants in COPD, but, given the association of COPD depression with anxiety symptoms, an SSRI or mirtazapine can be given. Benzodiazepines should be avoided, as they depress respiration. Pulmonary rehabilitation, based on activation and physical conditioning, along with an antidepressant, may be an effective approach, compared with medication alone. Cognitive behavioural therapy (CBT) and group educational interventions have been found to alleviate depression and anxiety symptoms and improve quality of life in patients with COPD (Kunik *et al.* 2007).

7.9.7 **Pain**

Where depression and pain coexist, treatment with both analgesics and antidepressants leads to better depression outcomes and lower reported pain than either given alone.

Key references

Alexopoulos GS (2005). Depression in the elderly. *The Lancet*, **365**, 1961–70.

Baldwin RC, Chiu E, Katona C, Graham N; under the auspices of the World Psychiatric Association Sections of Old Age Psychiatry and Affective Disorders (2002). *Guidelines on depression in older people: practising the evidence*. Martin Dunitz, London.

Banerjee S, Hellier J, Dewey M, *et al.* (2011). Sertraline or mirtazapine for depression in dementia (HTA-SADD): a randomised, multicentre, double-blind, placebo-controlled trial. *The Lancet*, **378**, 403–11.

Bower P, Kontopantelis E, Sutton A, *et al.* (2013). Influence of initial severity of depression on effectiveness of low intensity interventions: meta-analysis of individual patient data. *BMJ*, **346**, 540.

Brooke P and Bullock R (1999). Validation of the 6 item cognitive impairment test. *International Journal of Geriatric Psychiatry*, **14**, 936–40.

Castro VM, Clements CC, Murphy SN, *et al.* (2013). QT interval and antidepressant use: a cross-sectional study of electronic health records. *BMJ*, **346**, f288.

Dodd S, Horgan D, Malhi GS, Berk M (2005). To combine or not to combine? A literature review of antidepressant combination therapy. *Journal of Affective Disorders*,**89**, 1–11.

Gladsjo JA, Schuman CC, Evans JD, Peavy GM, Miller GW, Heaton RK (1999). Norms for letter and category fluency: demographic corrections for age, education, and ethnicity. *Assessment*, **6**, 147–78.

Goldberg JF and Thase ME (2013). Monoamine oxidase inhibitors revisited: what you should know. *Journal of Clinical Psychiatry*, **74**, 189–91.

Haney EM and Warden SJ (2009). Skeletal effects of serotonin (5-hydroxytryptamine) transporter inhibition: evidence from clinical studies. *Journal of Musculoskeletal and Neuronal Interactions*, **8**, 133–45.

Jin H, Shih PB, Golshan S, *et al.* (2013). Comparison of longer-term safety and effectiveness of 4 atypical antipsychotics in patients over age 40: a trial using equipoise-stratified randomization. *Journal of Clinical Psychiatry*, **74**, 10–18.

Jorge JRE, Moser DJ, Acion L, Robinson RG (2008). Treatment of vascular depression using repetitive transcranial magnetic stimulation. *Archives of General Psychiatry*, **65**, 268–76.

Karaiskos D, Pappa D, Tzavellas E, *et al.* (2013). Pregabalin augmentation of antidepressants in older patients with comorbid depression and generalized anxiety disorder—an open-label study. *International Journal of Geriatric Psychiatry*, **28**, 100–5.

Kok RM, Nolen WA, Heeren TJ (2009). Outcome of late-life depression after 3 years of sequential treatment. *Acta Psychiatrica Scandinavica*, **119**, 274–81.

Kok RM, Nolen WA, Heeren TJ (2012). Efficacy of treatment in older depressed patients: a systematic review and meta-analysis of double-blind randomized controlled trials with antidepressants. *Journal of Affective Disorders*, **141**, 103–15.

Kunik ME, Veazey C, Cully JA, *et al.* (2007). COPD education and cognitive behavioural therapy group treatment for clinically significant symptoms of depression and anxiety in COPD patients a randomized controlled trial. *Psychological Medicine*, **37**, 1–12.

Kvelde T, McVeigh KT, Toson B, *et al.* (2013). Depressive symptoms as a risk factor for falls in older people: systematic review and meta-analysis. *Journal of the American Geriatrics Society*, **61**, 694–706.

Lehmann SW and Lee J (2013). Lithium-associated hypercalcemia and hyperparathyroidism in the elderly: what do we know? *Journal of Affective Disorders*, **146**, 151–7.

Lotrich FE and Pollock BG (2005). Aging and clinical pharmacology: implications for antidepressants. *Journal of Clinical Pharmacology*, **45**, 1106–22.

Marriott A, Donaldson C, Tarrier N, Burns A (2000). Effectiveness of cognitive—behavioural family intervention in reducing the burden of care in carers of patients with Alzheimer's disease. *British Journal of Psychiatry*, **176**, 557–62.

McDermott CL and Gray SL (2012). Cholinesterase inhibitor adjunctive therapy for cognitive impairment and depressive symptoms in older adults with depression. *Annals of Pharmacotherapy*, **46**, 599–605.

Menza M, Dobkin RD, Marin H, *et al.* (2009). A controlled trial of antidepressants in patients with Parkinson disease and depression. *Neurology*, **72**, 886–92.

Montgomery S, Chatamra K, Pauer L, Whalen E, Baldinetti F (2008). Efficacy and safety of pregabalin in elderly people with generalised anxiety disorder. *British Journal of Psychiatry*, **193**, 389–94.

Mottram P, Wilson K, Strobl J (2006). Antidepressants for depressed elderly. *Cochrane Database of Systematic Reviews*, **1**, CD003491.

Nasreddine ZS, Phillips NA, Bédirian V, *et al.* (2005). The Montreal cognitive assessment (MoCA): a brief screening tool for mild cognitive impairment. *Journal of the American Geriatrics Society*, 53, 695–9.

National Institute for Health and Clinical Excellence (NICE) (2006). *Bipolar disorder: the management of bipolar disorder in adults, children and adolescents, in primary and secondary care*. Clinical guideline 38. NICE, London.

National Institute for Health and Clinical Excellence (NICE) (2009). *NICE clinical guideline 90. Depression: the treatment and management of depression in adults (partial update of NICE clinical guideline 23)*. NICE, London.

National Institute for Health and Clinical Excellence (NICE) (2009). *Depression with a chronic physical health problem*. Clinical guideline 91. NICE, London.

Nelson JC, Delucchi K, Schneider LS (2008). Efficacy of second generation antidepressants in late-life depression: a meta-analysis of the evidence. *American Journal of Geriatric Psychiatry*, **16**, 558–67.

Nelson JC and Papakostas GI (2009). Atypical antipsychotic augmentation in major depressive disorder: a meta-analysis of placebo-controlled randomized trials. *American Journal of Psychiatry*, **166**, 980–91.

Paranthaman R and Baldwin RC (2006). Treatments of psychiatric syndromes due to cerebrovascular disease. *International Review of Psychiatry*, **18**, 453–70.

Pinquart M, Duberstein PR, Lyness JM (2006). Treatments for later-life depressive conditions: a meta-analytic comparison of pharmacotherapy and psychotherapy. *American Journal of Psychiatry*, **163**, 1493–501.

Reynolds CF III, Dew MA, Pollock BG, *et al.* (2006). Maintenance treatment of major depression in old age. *New England Journal of Medicine*, **354**, 1130–8.

Reynolds CF III, Frank E, Perel JM, *et al.* (1999). Nortriptyline and interpersonal psychotherapy as maintenance therapies for recurrent major depression: a randomized controlled trial in patients older then 59 years. *Journal of the American Medical Association*, **281**, 39–45.

Richards JB, Papaioannou A, Adachi JD, *et al.*; for the Canadian Multicentre Osteoporosis Study (CaMos) Research Group (2007). Effect of selective serotonin reuptake inhibitors on the risk of fracture. *Archives of Internal Medicine*, **167**, 188–94.

Robinson RG, Jorge RE, Moser DJ, *et al.* (2008). Escitalopram and problem-solving therapy for prevention of post-stroke depression: a randomized controlled trial. *Journal of the American Medical Association*, **299**, 2391–400.

Romeo R, Knapp M, Hellier J, *et al.* (2013). Cost-effectiveness analyses for mirtazapine and sertraline in dementia: randomised controlled trial. *British Journal of Psychiatry*, **202**, 121–8.

Taylor D, Paton C, Kapur SR (2012). *The Maudsley prescribing guidelines*, 11th edition. Wiley-Blackwell, London.

Tedeschini E, Levkovitz Y, Iovieno N, Ameral VE, Nelson JC, Papakostas GI (2011). Efficacy of antidepressants for late-life depression: a meta-analysis and meta-regression of placebo-controlled randomized trials. *Journal of Clinical Psychiatry*, **72**, 1660–8.

Waldorff FB, Buss DV, Eckermann A, *et al.* (2012). Efficacy of psychosocial intervention in patients with mild Alzheimer's disease: the multicentre, rater blinded, randomised Danish Alzheimer Intervention Study (DAISY). *BMJ*, **345**, e4693.

Chapter 8

Depression in primary care

Key points

- Primary care is an important place for detecting late-life depression.
- Most suicides in older adults have had recent contact with primary care services.
- Case identification of depression is more effective when targeted toward those at most risk, for example, those with a chronic disease.
- There are several instruments which can be used to identify older people with depression, including those with depression plus dementia.
- There are important barriers which must be overcome for the successful detection and management of depression in later life.
- Collaborative care between primary and specialist care, utilizing a depression care manager, is more effective than usual care.

This chapter utilizes concepts and information from other chapters and adapts them to the context of primary care. Whether or not depression in primary care is under-recognized and under-treated continues to be debated, but primary care has a crucial role in detecting and treating late-life depressive disorder (see Box 8.1). Specialists see only a fraction of those affected by, or at risk of, depression. Chapter 4 has highlighted that older people who commit suicide have had little interaction with specialist services, but most have had contact with primary care, making this an important place for identifying those most at risk.

8.1 Case identification

The English National Institute for Health and Care Excellence (NICE, 2009) suggests a two-question screen for depression (see Box 8.2). Although highly sensitive (almost 100%), very short case detection instruments have low specificity and may not be sufficiently accurate for use in general practice (Mitchell and Coyne 2007). Chapter 5 of the NICE depression guideline CG90 (2009) has a detailed overview of case identification, the term now preferred to 'screening'. In relation to suicide, case identification of depression remains an important pathway for prevention.

The geriatric depression scale (GDS) has been developed specifically for older adults. It has 30 questions and is reproduced in the Appendix. It avoids questions which rely on physical symptoms and uses a simple yes/no format. It is meant to be self-administered, but rater assistance is acceptable. There are shorter versions, including a 15-item version

Box 8.1 Case identification in late-life depression (see Appendix)

Geriatric depression scale (GDS).
Hospital anxiety and depression scale (HADS).
Patient health questionnaire (PHQ-9).
World Health Organization well-being index.
Cornell scale for depression in dementia.

Box 8.2 NICE case identification questions for depression

- During the last month, have you often been bothered by feeling down, depressed, or hopeless?
- During the last month, have you often been bothered by having little interest or pleasure in doing things?

NICE (2009) *Depression: management of depression in primary and secondary care CG90.*

Box 8.3 The four most sensitive questions from the GDS*

- Are you basically satisfied with your life?
- Do you feel that your life is empty?
- Are you afraid that something bad is going to happen to you?
- Do you feel happy most of the time?

*A score of 2 or more indicates a probable depressive disorder.

and a 4-item one, using questions 1, 3, 8, and 9 (see Box 8.3). There is a GDS website with the various versions, bibliography, and translations into Chinese, Creole, Danish, Dutch, Farsi, French, French Canadian, German, Greek, Hebrew, Hindi, Hungarian, Icelandic, Italian, Japanese, Korean, Lithuanian, Malay, Portuguese, Russian, Russian Ukrainian, Spanish, Swedish, Thai, Turkish, Vietnamese, and Yiddish (<http://stanford.edu/~yesavage/GDS.html>). There are iPhone and Android apps for the GDS.

Despite its name, the hospital anxiety and depression scale (HADS) is also recommended for use in primary care and has been validated on older adults (Spinhoven et al. 1997). For case detection in primary care, it is the total score which best predicts the likelihood of depression. It takes about 5 minutes to complete, and its scores can be categorized as normal (0–7), mild (8–10), moderate (11–14), and severe (15–21), although research (Spinhoven et al. 1997) suggests that older adults with depression tend to score a little higher. It is copyrighted for commercial use and should be ordered from GL Assessment (<http://shop.gl-assessment.co.uk/home.php?cat=417&gclid=CKal7ZDI95cCFRNnQgodx23EDg>).

The patient health questionnaire (PHQ-9) (see Appendix 3) is widely used to screen for depression. It scores each of the nine DSM-IV criteria (now superseded by DSM-V but listed in Appendix) from '0' (not at all) to '3' (nearly every day). One or both of the first two questions should score at least '2' for depressive disorder to be likely. For a more definite diagnosis of major depression, five or more questions must be rated

Box 8.4 Improving recognition of late-life depressive disorder

- Remember that depressive disorder is not a normal part of ageing.
- Maintain awareness of the high frequency of depressive disorders.
- Become familiar with the core symptoms of depressive disorders.
- And do not discount treatment because there seems to be an understandable cause.
- And remember that the ageing process affects the presentation of depressive disorders.
- Give equal attention to physical and mental health.
- Develop skills for clinical interviewing of older persons.
- Avoid therapeutic nihilism ('nothing works').

as '2' or '3', except for question 9, for which any score above '0' is significant. In addition, question 10, functional impairment, is endorsed as at least 'somewhat difficult'. Patients can score themselves using the website: <http://www.patient.co.uk/doctor/patient-health-questionnaire-phq-9>.

The World Health Organization well-being index was developed as a rapid screening test for depression. The 1998 version (version 2) is reproduced in the Appendix and has been validated on people aged 50 and above (Bonsignore *et al.* 2001). A higher score indicates greater well-being. A score below 13 or a score of 0 or 1 to any of the five items suggests a high likelihood of depressive disorder.

The Cornell scale for detecting depression in dementia (see Appendix) utilizes observational data and is administered to the patient's caregiver (Alexopoulos *et al.* 1988). It takes a little longer (15–20 minutes) than other questionnaires but is more specific for depression in dementia than the other case identification instruments.

Given the importance of dementia as a differential diagnosis and as a common accompaniment to depression, detecting dementia is important. A short screening scale for dementia in primary care is the 6-item orientation-memory-concentration (OMC) test (Brooke and Bullock 2000).

Last, the importance of improving practitioners' 'mindset' to increase detection cannot be overstated. Suggestions are given in Box 8.4. Some of these are linked to barriers to detection, discussed later in the chapter.

8.2 Depression severity

Box 8.5 lists three severity measures which are straightforward to use. Probably the simplest is the PHQ which has been discussed. The PHQ can also serve as a guide to treatment (see Table 8.1) via scoring thresholds.

The HDRS covers 17 items and is observer-rated (Hamilton 1960), whereas the MADRAS (Montgomery and Äsberg 1979) is a mixture of self-report and observed behaviour. If copied for any use, other than individual research, the permission of the Royal College of Psychiatrists must be obtained. A 50% reduction in either scale is regarded as a treatment 'response', and remission is a score of <7 or <10, respectively.

Box 8.5 Severity rating scales (see Appendix)
The PHQ. 17-item Hamilton depression rating scale (HDRS). Montgomery-Äsberg depression rating scale (MADRAS).

Table 8.1 Severity scales with the PHQ-9

PHQ-9 score	Provisional diagnosis	Treatment recommendation
5-9	Minimal symptoms	Support, educate; see if worse; return in 1 month
10-14	Minor depression	Support, watchful waiting
	Dysthymia	Antidepressant or psychotherapy
	Major depression, *mild*	Antidepressant or psychotherapy
15-19	Major depression, *moderately severe*	Antidepressant or psychotherapy
≥20	Major depression, *severe*	Antidepressant <u>and</u> psychotherapy (especially if not improved on monotherapy)

8.3 Treatment principles

8.3.1 Deciding when to treat

There are concerns about medicalizing everyday problems in primary care, so the following three distinguishing characteristics are recommended to help come to a judgement about whether to treat depressive symptoms.

- *Duration:* symptoms are present for at least 2 weeks.
- *Lack of fluctuation:* symptoms occur on most days, most of the time.
- *Intensity:* of a degree that is definitely not normal for that individual and which interferes with function.

Figure 8.1 provides a framework for decision making when making a diagnosis in primary care.

8.3.2 Deciding on treatment

Table 8.1, linked to the PHQ, provides a simple way to link severity to treatment modality. Table 8.2 takes this a little further, linking types of depression to particular treatment. It is especially important in primary care to consider an organic depressive disorder (see Table 5.2) and to recognize psychotic depression. When treating older adults, general practitioners tend to select non-specific 'counselling', rather than the more evidence-based CBT (Katona and Shankar 2004). This may be a resource issue, but, increasingly, older people will expect an evidence-based psychological treatment.

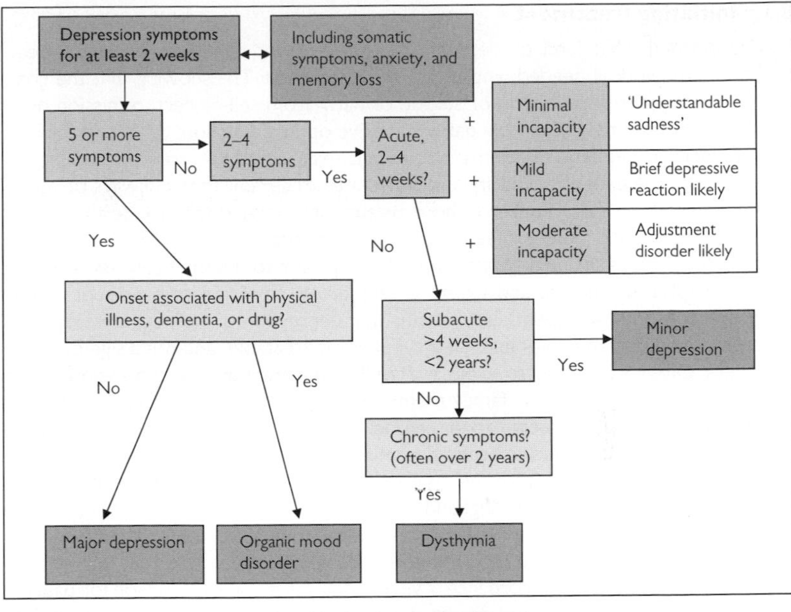

Figure 8.1 Depressive symptoms in later life: decision tree for diagnosis.

Table 8.2 Linking depression typology to treatment

Type of depression	Treatment modality
Psychotic depression	Combined antidepressant and antipsychotic drugs; sometimes electroconvulsive therapy—urgent referral indicated
Organic depressive disorder	Treat underlying medical disorder/change offending medication May still have to treat depressive syndrome
Severe (non-psychotic depression)	Combined antidepressant and psychological therapy—consider referral
Mild to moderate depressive episode	Antidepressant **or** psychological therapy (CBT, problem-solving, IPT, or brief psychodynamic psychotherapy)
Dysthymia	Antidepressant
Recent onset sub-threshold (minor) depression	Watchful waiting and support
Persistent sub-threshold (minor) depression	Antidepressant and support
Brief depression, grief reaction, and bereavement symptoms	Treat as for moderate depression if duration and intensity suggest intervention is indicated; otherwise, support and watchful waiting
Major depression with co-morbidity	Antidepressant, and consider optimum analgesia where relevant
Persistent minor depression with co-morbidity	Some evidence of the effectiveness of counselling or brief psychological treatment

8.3.3 **Initiating treatment**

Having decided what kind of depression is present and whether to initiate treatment, a framework is needed, and this is shown in Table 7.1, showing that the goals of treatment are: risk reduction-of suicide or harm from self-neglect; remission of all depressive symptoms; to help the patient achieve optimal function; to treat the whole person, including somatic problems; to prevent relapse and recurrence (discussed in Chapter 10). The patient's capacity and consent to treatment should always be ascertained (see Section 7.3.3.1). Throughout treatment, continue to educate the patient about depression and antidepressants, and offer support.

For older patients inclined to attribute all symptoms to a somatic illness, time set aside to explain the nature and extent of any actual physical illness present and its likely effects is time well spent. Emphasizing that depression is an illness can help clinical engagement, as can explaining that it is common, treatable, and not a sign of moral weakness. Often, it is helpful to explore a family's understanding of depression and of 'illness' in general. Sometimes, family members can unwittingly reinforce invalidism in depressed patients but, via education, can be helped to foster more adaptive coping. Patients must be encouraged to keep up as much activity and exercise as possible, perhaps keeping to a short 'programme' to encourage structure and purpose. Keeping to a balanced diet, avoiding overeating, and adhering to sleep hygiene are important. The latter includes avoiding caffeine drinks and alcohol near bedtime, using the bedroom for sleeping only, and keeping to a regular night-time routine.

Encouraging treatment concordance is vital, as the most common reason for patients not getting better is that the treatment is not being taken properly or not at all (see Box 7.3). Patients often need reassurance that antidepressants are not addictive and that depression is not 'senility' or a harbinger of dementia. They need to be warned not to expect immediate results. Commonly occurring side effects should be explained.

8.3.4 **The organization of treatment and support**

In England, the process of depression management is guided by the stepped care process (NICE 2009) (see Figure 8.2). Steps 1 to 2 are largely the domain of primary care. Step 3 may be in primary care, with support from specialist mental health services or, in the English NHS, via the Improving Access to Psychological Therapies initiative (IAPT, <http://www.iapt.nhs.uk/>). The IAPT initiative facilitates both low- and high-intensity treatments, mainly within the CBT model. Knowing when to refer for specialist advice is important (see Box 8.6).

Offering support is not doing nothing. Combined with empathy and understanding, it is a powerful therapeutic tool in depression.

8.4 **Barriers to treatment**

Barriers to accessing help for depression in primary care fall under the headings of patient-related, practitioner-related, organizational, and societal (see Table 8.3). Older people, poor people, and minority populations can be especially disadvantaged (Unützer *et al.* 1999). Ageism is a hidden barrier ('what's the point of treating depression at her age?'). No one sets out to be ageist, but honest self-scrutiny is needed to guard against it.

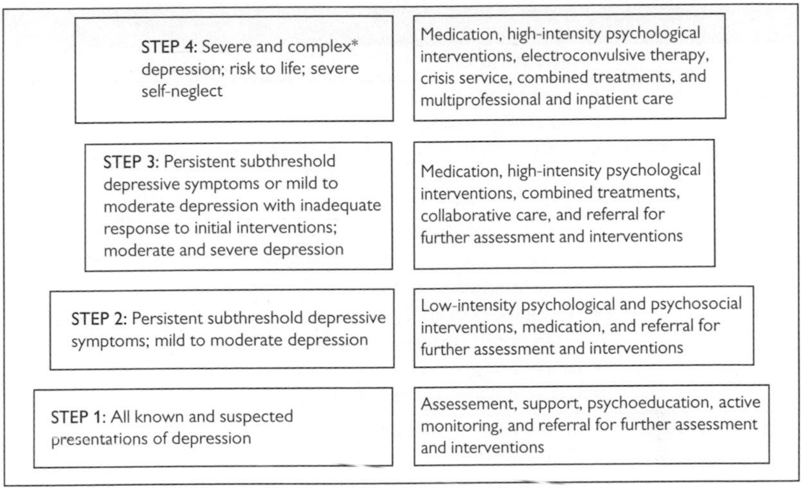

STEP 4: Severe and complex* depression; risk to life; severe self-neglect	Medication, high-intensity psychological interventions, electroconvulsive therapy, crisis service, combined treatments, and multiprofessional and inpatient care
STEP 3: Persistent subthreshold depressive symptoms or mild to moderate depression with inadequate response to initial interventions; moderate and severe depression	Medication, high-intensity psychological interventions, combined treatments, collaborative care, and referral for further assessment and interventions
STEP 2: Persistent subthreshold depressive symptoms; mild to moderate depression	Low-intensity psychological and psychosocial interventions, medication, and referral for further assessment and interventions
STEP 1: All known and suspected presentations of depression	Assessement, support, psychoeducation, active monitoring, and referral for further assessment and interventions

Figure 8.2 NICE stepped care model of depression treatment.

* Complex means not responsive or inadequately responsive to multiple treatment trials, psychotic depression, or significant co-morbidity or psychosocial factors.

National Institute for Health and Clinical Excellence (2009) CG 90 Depression: the treatment and management of depression in adults. London: NICE. Available from http://guidance.nice.org.uk/CG90 Reproduced with permission. This material is accurate at the time of going to press.

Box 8.6 Referring for specialist advice

- When the diagnosis in doubt (e.g. is this dementia?).
- When depression is severe, as evidenced by:
  - Psychotic symptoms.
  - Severe risk to health because of failure to eat or drink.
  - Suicide risk.
- Complex therapy is indicated (for example in cases with medical co-morbidity).
- When therapy fails (depending on local criteria this may be after two antidepressants have been tried from different classes).
- Complex psychosocial factors.

In primary care, improving training about depression is probably the best way to start removing barriers.

8.5 **Collaborative care**

The collaborative care model has been developed to improve outcomes of depression in primary care. The components are a depression care manager (usually a nurse, psychologist, or social worker) who coordinates the care, including medication concordance, supervised by a psychiatrist. Medication is provided by the general

Table 8.3 Barriers to consider in primary care	
Factors	Possible barriers
Patient-related	• Somatization • Fear of stigmatization • Negative beliefs about antidepressant medication (for example, that they are addictive) • False normalization of depression
Practitioner-related	• Poor consultation skills • Ageism • False normalization of depression • 'Therapeutic nihilism' • Attribution of depression to societal ills • Lack of confidence and/or experience in treatments • Blinkered approach (seeing everything as either physical or mental)
Organizational	• Separation of mental health and medical services • Poor coordination of services • Lack of appropriate services (for example, psychological interventions) • Low reimbursement rates for psychotropic medication (in some countries)
Societal	• Lack of legislation regarding age discrimination

practitioner. Regular review can occur by face-to-face interview or telephone contact. The `IMPACT' study of older adults conducted in the United States is the largest to date (Unützer *et al.* 2002). A total of 1,801 depressed primary care patients (major depression, 17%; dysthymia, 30%; or both, 53%) were randomized to either a depression manager or usual care. There was a choice of problem-solving treatment (PST) or an antidepressant (prescribed by the general practitioner). At 12 months, 45% of intervention patients achieved a 50% reduction in symptoms, compared to 19% of usual care subjects. Another large study from the United States Prevention of Suicide in Primary Care Elderly Collaborative Trial (PROSPECT), using a similar model, found some effect in reducing suicidal thinking (Bruce *et al.* 2004). In the UK, this model has also been shown to be effective (Chew-Graham *et al.* 2007). In addition, the use of a collaborative care approach to the management of depressed residents in nursing homes has been shown to improve outcomes (Llewellyn-Jones *et al.* 1999). Importantly, the PROSPECT collaborative care model in primary care has been shown to reduce mortality in those with major depression, compared to usual care (by up to a quarter), perhaps because of its positive impact on holistic care and careful monitoring of suicidal thinking (Gallo *et al.* 2013).

Key references

Alexopoulos GS, Abrams RC, Shamoian CA (1988). Cornell scale for depression in dementia. *Biological Psychiatry*, **23**, 271–84.

Bonsignore M, Barkow K, Jessen F, Heun R (2001). Validity of the five-item WHO well-being index (WHO-5) in an elderly population. *European Archives of Psychiatry and Clinical Neurosciemces*, **251** (Suppl. 2), II/27–II/31.

Brooke P and Bullock R (1999). Validation of the 6 item cognitive impairment test. *International Journal of Geriatric Psychiatry*, **14**, 936–40.

Bruce ML, Have TRT, Reynolds CF, *et al.* (2004). Reducing suicidal ideation and depressive symptoms in depressed older primary care patients: a randomized controlled trial. *Journal of the American Medical Association*, **291**, 1081–91.

Chew-Graham CA, Lovell K, Roberts C, *et al.* (2007). Implementation of the collaborative care model for the management of depression in the elderly in the UK. *British Journal of General Practice*, **57**, 364–70.

Gallo JJ, Morales KH, Bogner HR, *et al.* (2013). Long term effect of depression care management on mortality in older adults: follow-up of cluster randomized clinical trial in primary care. *BMJ*, **346**, f2570.

Hamilton M (1960). A rating scale for depression. *Journal of Neurology, Neurosurgery & Psychiatry*, **23**, 56–62.

Iliffe S, Gould MM, Mitchley S. (1994). Evaluation of brief screening instruments for depression, dementia and problem drinking in general practice. *British Journal of General Practice*, **44**, 503–7.

Katona CLE and Shankar KK (2004). Depression in old age. *Reviews in Clinical Gerontology*, **14**, 283–306.

Llewellyn-Jones RH, Baikie KA, Smithers H, Cohen J, Snowdon J, Tennant CC (1999). Multifaceted shared care intervention for late life depression in residential care: randomised controlled trial. *BMJ*, **319**, 676–82.

Mitchell AJ and Coyne JC (2007). Do ultra-short screening instruments accurately detect depression in primary care: a pooled analysis and meta-analysis of 22 studies. *British Journal of General Practice*, **57**, 144–51.

Montgomery SA and Äsberg M (1979). A new depression scale designed to be sensitive to change. *British Journal of Psychiatry*, **134**, 382–9.

National Institute for Health and Clinical Excellence (NICE) (2009). *NICE clinical guideline 90. Depression: the treatment and management of depression in adults (partial update of NICE clinical guideline 23)*. NICE, London.

Spinhoven PH, Ormel J, Sloekers PPA, Kempen G (1997). A validation study of the Hospital Anxiety and Depression Scale (HADS) in different groups of Dutch subjects. *Psychological Medicine*, **27**, 363–70.

Unützer J, Katon W, Sullivan M, Miranda J (1999). Treating depressed older adults in primary care: narrowing the gap between efficacy and effectiveness. *The Millbank Quarterly*, **77**, 225–56.

Unützer J, Katon W, Callahan C, *et al.* (2002). Collaborative care management of late-life depression in the primary care setting. *Journal of the American Medical Association*, **288**, 2836–45.

Zigmond AS and Snaith RP (1983). The Hospital Anxiety And Depression Scale. *Acta Psychiatrica Scandinavica*, **67**, 361–70.

Chapter 9

Prognosis

Key points
• Depression in later life is a recurrent disorder. • Mortality may be increased in late-life depression. • There is evidence that depression is a risk factor for dementia in later life.

9.1 **Outcome in naturalistic studies**

In all age groups, depressive disorder is a condition prone to recurrence, which is why its management as a chronic (long-term) health condition makes sense. However, naturalistic studies (that is studies outside of controlled trials) provide evidence that the prognosis under specialist care is better than that seen in the community where there may be considerable treatment variability or no treatment at all (Beekman *et al.* 2002). Why this is so is unclear, but there are likely to be differences in risk factors, levels of detection, adequacy of treatment, and medical co-morbidity, all of which can influence outcome.

As regards comparative outcome, Mitchell and Subramanian (2005) reviewed the literature finding that episodes of depression remitted as well in later life as in other age groups, but with a greater risk of relapse in older people. This was linked to two factors: age of onset (recurrent depression from earlier life was associated with a poorer prognosis) and medical co-morbidity (associated with a later onset and worse prognosis). This suggests that interventions in the continuation and maintenance phases of treatment (see Chapter 10) are especially important in late-life depression.

Compared to those without depression, patients identified by screening as depressed, whilst on a medical ward, have a worse prognosis in terms of increased mortality and an increased likelihood of further care in a rehabilitation facility or a nursing home. In an acute hospital setting, an intervention package, comprising problem-solving, brief support, and referral to relevant support agencies, did reduce depressive symptomatology but not length of stay (Baldwin *et al.* 2004).

9.2 **Mortality**

A number of studies suggest that having depression is associated with an increased death rate in older adults. Blazer *et al.* (2001) though found that this effect was markedly attenuated, if not abolished, once factors, such as chronic disease, health habits, cognitive impairment, functional impairment, and level of social support, were taken

Box 9.1 Possible mechanisms to explain an increased mortality in depressive disorder

- Medical co-morbidity.
- Illness effects (e.g. inertia from psychomotor retardation).
- Behavioural factors:
  - Reduced physical activity.
  - Poor diet.
  - Smoking.
  - Alcohol misuse.
  - Poor health self-maintenance.
- Poor adherence to prescribed medication.
- Effects from occult illness (e.g. carcinoma not evident at diagnosis).
- Possible treatment effects (e.g. tricyclic drugs and cardiotoxicity).
- Biological factors (e.g. raised cortisol from chronic depression).

into account, making this a controversial subject. Also controversial is the extent to which suicide contributes to an increase in mortality.

Several mechanisms to explain why depression may increase mortality in depressive disorders have been proposed (see Box 9.1). These included the effects of co-morbid physical illness; occult illness (e.g. an unsuspected carcinoma); indirect effects of depression (e.g. pneumonia triggered by psychomotor retardation); treatment effects (e.g. some of the older tricyclic antidepressants are thought to be cardiotoxic); and biological effects (e.g. raised cortisol level). To these can be added behavioural factors (lack of exercise, smoking, alcohol misuse, and limited activity); poorer health self-maintenance (e.g. not going for blood pressure checks); and the consequences of the fact that depressed patients are less likely to adhere to medication for medical conditions.

9.3 **Prognostic factors**

Predictive factors may be divided into **general factors** and **specific clinical features of the illness**. Box 9.2 lists some of the poor outcome factors, subdivided by illness features and general factors. Adversity includes chronic stress associated with a poor environment; crime and poverty; becoming a victim of crime; poor social support; and the development of serious physical ill health. Surprisingly, few features of the illness itself can be linked definitively to a poor prognosis. The literature suggests that the following are important: a slow or incomplete recovery; three or more previous episodes; severity of initial depression; longer duration from onset (especially if over 2 years); and the presence of organic cerebral pathology.

9.4 **Dementia**

Although depression will sometimes be an early symptom of dementia, recent epidemiological evidence shows that depression is itself a risk factor for later dementia, both vascular and Alzheimer's disease. Pragmatically, a first depressive episode which

Box 9.2 Poor outcome factors

Illness—clinical features

- Slower initial recovery
- More severe initial depression
- Duration more than 2 years
- Number of previous episodes (three and above increases risk)
- Chronic symptomatology with residual symptoms
- Psychotic depression
- Extensive disease of deep white matter and/or basal ganglia grey matter (vascular depression)
- Underlying organic brain disease (for example, dementia)

General factors

- Chronic stress associated with poor environment, crime, and poverty
- A new physical illness
- Becoming a victim of crime
- Poor perceived (even if not objectively lacking) social support

occurred within 10 years of the onset of dementia is likely to have been an early symptom of it. As a risk factor, in one recent study, there was a gradient of increased risk from those who experienced depression in earlier life only (lowest risk but still increased relative to no depression), to those with depression only in later life, and to those who had both earlier depression and later life depression, the latter having a threefold raised risk (Barnes *et al.* 2012). This should, however, be kept in perspective—the great majority of people who have had depression do not develop dementia.

Key references

Baldwin R, Pratt H, Goring H, Marriott A, Roberts C (2004). Does a nurse-led mental health liaison service for older people reduce psychiatric morbidity in acute general medical wards? A randomised controlled trial. *Age and Ageing*, **33**, 472–8.

Barnes DE, Yaffe K, Byers AL, McCormick M, Schaefer C, Whitmer RA (2012). Midlife vs late-life depressive symptoms and risk of dementia: differential effects for Alzheimer disease and vascular dementia. *Archives of General Psychiatry*, **69**, 493–8.

Beekman AT, Geerlings SW, Deeg DJ, *et al.* (2002). The natural history of late-life depression. A 6-year prospective study in the community. *Archives of General Psychiatry*, **59**, 605–11.

Blazer D, Hybels C, Pieper C (2001). The association of depression and mortality in elderly persons: a case for multiple independent pathways. *Journal of Gerontology: Medical Sciences*, **56A**, M505–9.

Mitchell AJ and Subramaniam H (2005). Prognosis of depression in old age compared to middle age: a systematic review of comparative studies. *American Journal of Psychiatry*, **162**, 1588–601.

Chapter 10

Prevention

Key points

- The primary prevention of late-life depression may be a realistic goal.
- Secondary prevention of depressive disorder has a strong evidence base.

The phases of depression treatment are illustrated in Figure 10.1 (Frank *et al.* 1991). The acute phase has been covered. Continuation treatment follows remission and is aimed at preventing a return of symptoms (relapse). It is measured in months. Maintenance treatment aims to prevent future depressive episodes (recurrence) and is measured in years.

10.1 Primary prevention

The primary prevention of depression can be divided into universal, selective, and indicated. Universal prevention acts to minimize risk factors at the population level, as in screening for hypertension. In mental health, this is costly and of unproven benefit. Selective intervention targets only that portion of the population with identified risk factors. In mental health, examples include several chronic medical conditions known to be associated with a high risk of depression. Selective primary prevention has been shown to be effective for stroke and macular degeneration but not hip fracture (summarized by Baldwin 2010). A third type of primary prevention, indicated prevention, targets people who already manifest some symptoms of the designated disorder but at an early or sub-syndromal stage. In the context of this chapter, the example is sub-threshold depression which can be screened for in settings such as primary care.

Schoevers *et al.* (2006) discuss the evidence for selective and indicated prevention in terms of likely clinical and economic benefit and concluded that the indicated approach was preferable. In other words, because sub-threshold depression is such a risk factor for major depression, an approach which targets interventions to those with sub-threshold depression is likely to prove effective. van't Veer-Tazelaar *et al.* (2009) found that a programme of care progressively stepped through various interventions in those with sub-threshold depression (i.e. an indicated prevention approach) resulted in a halving of the rate of conversion to major depression at 12 months.

The PROSPECT (Prevention of Suicide in Primary Care Elderly—Collaborative Trial) mentioned earlier (see Chapter 4) enrolled 598 subjects, 396 with major depression and 202 with sub-threshold symptoms. Treatment, using either an SSRI or interpersonal

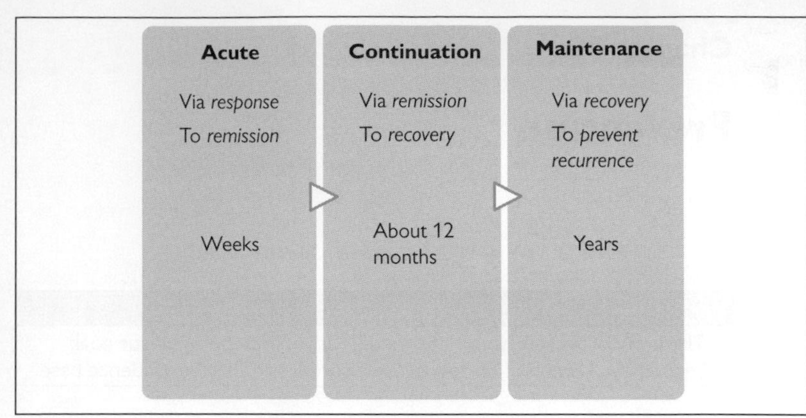

Figure 10.1 Conceptualization of phases of treatment in depression

therapy, was effective in reducing depressive symptoms in major depression as well as suicidal ideation in minor depression, an effect which was sustained (Alexopoulos *et al.* 2009).

10.2 **Secondary prevention**

This refers to preventing future recurrences of depression or relapse soon after an episode. Continuation treatment typically lasts between 6 and 12 months, with old age psychiatrists tending to recommend the longer side of this interval. A pragmatic approach is to recommend a minimum of 12 months' continuation treatment for a first episode, 24 months for a second, and at least 3 years for three or more episodes. In psychotic depression, antipsychotic medication is usually continued for 4–6 months, with gradual withdrawal if the patient remains well.

Patients remitted from depressive disorder should be followed up. Kiosses and Alexopoulos (2013) have shown that patients who developed even a few recurrent symptoms in the first 6 months after recovery had a much shorter time to relapse. Further, the longer the period of sub-threshold symptoms, the higher the recurrence rate at 2 years (Kiosses and Alexopoulos 2013).

Following recovery, there is considerable evidence that maintenance medication is effective in preventing a recurrence of depression. This has been demonstrated for tricyclic antidepressants, SSRIs, psychological treatments combined with antidepressants and lithium. As with other age groups, the general rule is to keep the antidepressant dose as close as possible to the one which the patient was taking on recovery ('the dose that got you well keeps you well').

Key references

Alexopoulos GS, Reynolds III CF, Bruce ML, *et al.* (2009). Reducing suicidal ideation and depression in older primary care patients: 24-month outcomes of the PROSPECT study. *American Journal of Psychiatry*, **166**, 882–90.

Baldwin RC (2010). Preventing late-life depression: a clinical update. *International Psychogeriatrics*, **22** (Special Issue 08), 1216–24.

Frank E, Prien RF, Jarrett RB, *et al.* (1991). Conceptualization and rationale for consensus definitions of terms in major depressive disorder. Remission, recovery, relapse, and recurrence. *Archives of General Psychiatry*, **48**, 851–5.

Kiosses DN and Alexopoulos GS (2013). The prognostic significance of subsyndromal symptoms emerging after remission of late-life depression. *Psychological Medicine*, **43**, 341–50.

Schoevers RA, Smit F, Deeg DJH, *et al.* (2006). Prevention of late-life depression in primary care: do we know where to begin? *American Journal of Psychiatry*, **163**, 1611–21.

van't Veer-Tazelaar PJ, van Marwijk HMJ, van Oppen P, *et al.* (2009). Stepped-care prevention of anxiety and depression in late life: a randomized controlled trial. *Archives of General Psychiatry*, **66**, 297–304.

Chapter 11

Resources

There is wealth of information to help patients, practitioners, and caregivers. The internet, in particular, has led to an explosion of potential sources of help, although the quality cannot always be guaranteed. This chapter contains merely a fraction of what is available from reliable sources.

11.1 Practitioner resources

11.1.1 Treatment of depression

An Expert Consensus guideline from the US, led by Dr George Alexopoulos and colleagues, has been published (Alexopoulos *et al.* 2001) and is outlined on <http://www.psychguides.com/depressive-disorders-in-older-patients/>, although the full professional guidance (link to 'experts, and contents pages from the guidelines') must be purchased.

The Sections of Old Age Psychiatry and Affective Disorder of the World Health Organization have produced a guideline book for late-life depression (Baldwin *et al.* 2002). Google, with permission of the publisher, has sample chapters. Go to Google Books search <http://books.google.com/>, and type in 'guidelines on depression in older people' (you may need to register with Google).

A shorter guideline from the Faculty of Old Age Psychiatry of the UK Royal College of Psychiatrists (Baldwin *et al.* 2003) is available via the website of *International Journal of Geriatric Psychiatry*. Those with journal access rights (for example, Athens password) can download it.

Consensus Guidelines for Assessment and Management of Depression in the Elderly Faculty of Psychiatry of Old Age, NSW Branch, Royal Australian and New Zealand College of Psychiatrists is a short guide with a number of useful algorithms, including ones on assessment (including suicide risk evaluation) and treatment (<http://www0.health.nsw.gov.au/pubs/2001/depression_elderly.html>).

The Canadian Coalition for Seniors' Mental Health (CCSMH) provides detailed guidelines on three relevant aspects: Assessment and Treatment of Depression; The Assessment and Treatment of Mental Health Issues in Long Term Care Homes (with a focus on mood and behavioural symptoms); and the Assessment of Suicide Risk and Prevention of Suicide. These are freely available (subject to registering on the website) by following the tab CCSMH Tools for Healthcare Providers at <http://www.ccsmh.ca/>.

The British Association of Psychopharmacology (BAP) has a detailed evidence-based guideline on depression from the *Journal of Psychopharmacology* (Anderson *et al.*

2008) and is accessible online at <http://www.bap.org.uk/docsbycategory.php?docCatID=2>.

In the UK, the National Institute for Health and Care Excellence (NICE) (<http://www.nice.org.uk/>) has a number of relevant guidelines. These have been referenced already (see Chapter 7, for example) and include unipolar depression (CG 90 and 91), electroconvulsive treatment (ECT) (TA 59, a technology appraisal), and self-harm (CG 16).

CANMAT (Canadian Network for Mood and Anxiety Treatments) is a not-for-profit research organization, linking health care professionals from across Canada who have a special interest in mood and anxiety disorders. Although not specifically for later life, the guidance covers much more than medication management (<http://www.canmat.org/resources/CANMAT%20Depression%20Guidelines%202009.pdf>).

Health Net provides an overview of guidelines on depressive disorder, covering diagnosis, interventions, and resources. There is a short section on older people (<https://www.healthnet.com/static/general/unprotected/pdfs/national/policies/MajorDepression.pdf>).

11.1.2 **Bipolar disorder**

Although bipolar disorder is not a primary focus of this book, depression is a major cause of disability in patients with bipolar disorder. The BAP has published a guideline on bipolar disorder (2009) which is accessible online (http://www.bap.org.uk/pdfs/Bipolar_guidelines.pdf).

The National Institute for Health and Care Excellence (NICE) (CG 38) also has guidance which is again downloadable (<http://www.nice.org.uk/nicemedia/live/10990/30193/30193.pdf>).

The Cochrane Collaboration publishes detailed reviews from research and makes evidence-based recommendations. A review of antidepressants in the elderly was published in 2009 but seems to include research only from papers in the 1990s and, therefore, misses some newer antidepressants.

(<http://www.thecochranelibrary.com/details/browseReviews/576825/Depressive-disorders--major-depression.html>).

11.2 **Patient education material**

The GDS can be completed online via the GDS website <http://www.stanford.edu/~yesavage> (follow links to testing page).

The American Association for Geriatric Psychiatry has material on depression available through the website of The Geriatric Mental Health Foundation (GMHF): A Guide to Mental Wellness in Older Age: Recognizing and Overcoming Depression (A Depression Recovery Toolkit) and Depression in Late Life: Not a Natural Part of Aging (also available in Spanish) (<http://www.gmhfonline.org/gmhf/consumer/depression.html>). The GMHF website also contains a number of useful links to other North American organizations.

Also from the United States, there is an information booklet for patients and caregivers (<http://www.psychguides.com/guides/depressive-disorder-in-older-patients/>).

CANMAT, mentioned in the previous section, also offers brief patient-oriented information about a range of common mental disorders, including depression in later life (<http://www.canmat.org/di-depression.php>).

The Black Dog Institute is an educational, research, clinical, and community-oriented facility based in Australia, dedicated to improving understanding, diagnosis, and treatment of mood disorders. It produces a number of fact sheets, including one on depression in old age (<http://www.blackdoginstitute.org.au/docs/DepressioninOlderPeople.pdf>).

In the UK, the Royal College of Psychiatrists produces patient information, again including one on depression in later life (<http://www.rcpsych.ac.uk/pdf/DOA.pdf>).

Age UK is a charity covering many aspects of life as an older person. It provides fact sheets on depression (<http://www.ageuk.org.uk/search1/?keyword=depression&nation=ageuk_en-GB>).

11.3 **Organizations for patients**

Cruse Bereavement Care
PO Box 800, Richmond, Surrey TW9 1RG, UK
Web: <http://www.crusebereavementcare.org.uk/>
Tel: 0844 477 9400
Email: helpline@cruse.org.uk

Bipolar UK (formerly the Manic Depressive Fellowship)
11 Belgrave Road, London SW1V 1RB, UK
Web: <http://www.mdf.org.uk/>
Tel: 0207 931 6480

MIND (National Association for Mental Health)
15–19 Broadway, Stratford, London E15 4BQ, UK Web: <http://www.mind.org.uk/>
Tel: 0300 123 3393
Email: contact@mind.org.uk
Provides a variety of information, including generic leaflets on depression and drugs to treat depression in a range of languages.

Depression Alliance
20 Great Dover Street, London SE1 4LX, UK Web: <http://www.depressionalliance.org>Tel: 0845 123 23 20
Email: information@depressionalliance.org
Provides information, support, and understanding to those who are affected by depression.

Age UK (formerly Help The Aged)
Tavis House, 1–6 Tavistock Square, London WC1H 9NA, UK
Web: <http://www.ageuk.org.uk/>
Tel: 0800 169 65 65
Email: via the 'Contact Us' tab

SANE
First Floor Cityside House, 40 Adler Street, London E1 1EE, UK
Web: <http://www.sane.org.uk>
Tel: 0845 767 8000
Email: via 'Contact us' tab
Works to improve quality of life for anyone affected by mental illness and provides free help.

11.4 **Self-help material**

The British Association of Behavioural and Cognitive Psychotherapies (BABCP)
Imperial House, Hornby Street, Bury BL9 5BN, UK
Web: <http://www.babcp.com>
Tel: 0161 705 4304
Email: babcp@babcp.com
The BABCP is the lead organization for CBT in the UK. Its website provides a guide to CBT as well as advice about finding a therapist. The organization maintains a register of qualified practitioners. It has some free online CBT resources but not specifically for late-life depression.

Oxford Cognitive Therapy Centre (OCTC)
Warneford Hospital, Oxford OX3 7JX, UK
Web: <http://www.octc.co.uk>
Tel: 01865 738 816
Email: octc@oxfordhealth.nhs.uk
The website gives details of how to order a number of educational and self-help booklets with a CBT approach for a range of conditions including depression.

Ultrasis
Web: <http://www.ultrasis.com>
Ultrasis produces interactive, computer-based CBT programmes for health care professionals, corporations, and consumers, including *Beating the Blues* (<http://www.beatingtheblues.co.uk/>) which has been endorsed for mild-to-moderate depression by the National Institute for Health and Clinical Excellence (NICE) (2006, technology assessment 97 <http://guidance.nice.org.uk/TA97/Guidance/pdf/English>).

Key references

Alexopoulos GS, Katz IR, Reynolds CF, Carpenter D, Docherty JP (2001). *The expert consensus guideline series: pharmacotherapy of depressive disorders in older patients. Postgraduate Medicine Special Report* (October), pp. 1–86. Expert Knowledge Systems, LLC, McGraw-Hill Healthcare Information Programs, Minneapolis.

Anderson IM, Ferrier IN, Baldwin R, *et al.*; on behalf of the Consensus Meeting; endorsed by the British Association for Psychopharmacology (2008). Evidence-based guidelines for treating depressive disorders with antidepressants: a revision of the 2000 British Association for Psychopharmacology guidelines. *Journal of Psychopharmacology*, **22**, 343–96.

Baldwin RC, Anderson D, Black S, *et al.*; Faculty of Old Age Psychiatry Working Group, Royal College of Psychiatrists (2003). Guideline for the management of late-life depression in primary care. *International Journal of Geriatric Psychiatry*, **18**, 829–38.

Baldwin RC, Chiu E, Katona C, Graham N (2002). *Guidelines on depression in older people: practising the evidence*. Martin Dunitz, London. ISBN 1841841269.

National Institute for Health and Clinical Excellence (NICE) (2003). *The clinical effectiveness and cost effectiveness of electroconvulsive therapy (ECT) for depressive illness, schizophrenia, catatonia and mania TA59*. National Institute for Health and Clinical Excellence, London.

National Institute for Health and Clinical Excellence (NICE) (2004). *Self-harm: the short-term physical and psychological management and secondary prevention of self-harm in primary and secondary care, CG016*. National Institute for Health and Clinical Excellence, London.

National Institute for Health and Clinical Excellence (NICE) (2006). *Health technology assessment No 97. Depression and anxiety—computerised cognitive behavioural therapy (CCBT)*. National Institute for Health and Clinical Excellence, London.

National Institute for Health and Clinical Excellence (NICE) (2006). *NICE clinical guideline 38. Bipolar disorder: the management of bipolar disorder in adults, children and adolescents, in primary and secondary care*. National Institute for Health and Clinical Excellence, London.

National Institute for Health and Clinical Excellence (NICE) (2009). *Depression: management of depression in adults, CG23*. National Institute for Health and Clinical Excellence, London.

General reading

Alexopoulos GS (2005). Depression in the elderly. *The Lancet*, **365**, 1961–70.

Baldwin RC, Chiu E, Katona C, Graham N (2002). *Guidelines on depression in older people: practising the evidence*. Under the auspices of the World Psychiatric Association Sections of Old Age Psychiatry and Affective Disorders. Martin Dunitz, London.

Blazer DG (2003). Depression in late life: review and commentary. *Journal of Gerontology: Medical Sciences*, **58A**, 249–65.

Katona CLE and Shankar KK (2004). Depression in old age. *Reviews in Clinical Gerontology*, **14**, 283–306.

Taylor D, Paton C, Kerwin R (2007). *The Maudsley prescribing guidelines*, 9th edition. Informa Health care, London.

Unützer J (2007). Late-life depression. *New England Journal of Medicine*, **357**, 2269–76.

WPA/PTD Educational Program on Depressive Disorders Module 1 Overview and Fundamental Aspects Module 3: Depressive Disorders in Older Persons. Available online at: <http://www.wpanet.org/education/ed-program-guidelines.shtml>.

Appendix 1

The sample rating scales

Table A1.1 Sample rating scales used in the assessment of depression in later life

Rating scale	Key features	Administrator	Time taken (min)
Geriatric depression scale	Available in 30-, 15-, and 4-item versions; easy to administer; available online; many translations	Patient or patient-assisted	10
Patient health questionnaire (PHQ-9)	Uses criteria from DSM-IV; brief and useful as primary care screen	Patient	5
The World Health Organization well-being index	Only five questions; brief primary care screen; scoring a little complicated; validated in older people	Patient	5
Cornell scale for depression in dementia	Only validated scale for depression in dementia; takes more time than a screening questionnaire	Clinician via carers or other observers	15–20
Hamilton depression rating scale (HDRS)	Widely used in clinical trials; requires knowledge of mental health; perhaps overly focussed on somatic symptoms	Clinician	15
Montgomery and Äsberg depression rating scale (MADRAS)	Widely used in clinical trials; non-specialist; sensitive to change	Clinician	15

Key references

Alexopoulos GS, Abrams RC, Shamoian CA (1988). Cornell scale for depression in dementia. *Biological Psychiatry*, **23**, 271–84.

Bonsignore M, Barkow K, Jessen F, Heun R (2001). Validity of the five-item WHO Well-Being Index (WHO-5) in an elderly population. *European Archives of Psychiatry and Clinical Neuroscience*, **251** (Suppl 2), II/27–II/31.

Hamilton M (1960). A rating scale for depression. *Journal of Neurology, Neurosurgery & Psychiatry*, **23**, 56–62.

Kroenke K and Spitzer RL (2002). The PHQ-9: a new depression and diagnostic severity measure. *Psychiatric Annals*, **32**, 509–21

Montgomery SA and Äsberg M (1979). A new depression scale designed to be sensitive to change. *British Journal of Psychiatry*, **134**, 382–9.

The sample rating scales

Key references

Appendix 2

The geriatric depression scale

Table A2.1 Sample sheet rating
Instructions: choose the best answer for how you have felt over the past **week**.
1. **Are you basically satisfied with your life?** No 2. **Have you dropped many of your activities and interests?** Yes 3. **Do you feel your life is empty?** Yes 4. **Do you often get bored?** Yes 5. Are you hopeful about the future? No 6. Are you bothered by thoughts you can't get out of your head? Yes 7. **Are you in good spirits most of the time?** No 8. **Are you afraid something bad is going to happen to you?** Yes 9. **Do you feel happy most of the time?** No 10. **Do you often feel helpless?** Yes 11. Do you often get restless and fidgety? Yes 12. **Do you prefer to stay at home, rather than going out and doing new things?** Yes 13. Do you frequently worry about the future? Yes 14. **Do you feel you have more problems with your memory than most?** Yes 15. **Do you think it is wonderful to be alive now?** No 16. Do you often feel down-hearted and blue (sad)? Yes 17. **Do you feel pretty worthless the way you are?** Yes 18. Do you worry a lot about the past? Yes 19. Do you find life very exciting? No 20. Is it hard for you to start on new projects (plans)? Yes 21. **Do you feel full of energy?** No 22. **Do you feel that your situation is hopeless?** Yes 23. **Do you think most people are better off (in their lives) than you are?** Yes 24. Do you frequently get upset over little things? Yes 25. Do you frequently feel like crying? Yes 26. Do you have trouble concentrating? Yes 27. Do you enjoy getting up in the morning? No 28. Do you prefer to avoid social gatherings (get-togethers)? Yes 29. Is it easy for you to make decisions? No 30. Is your mind as clear as it used to be? No
Notes: (1) Answers refer to responses which score '1'; (2) bracketed phrases refer to alternative ways of expressing the questions; (3) questions in bold comprise the 15-item version. Suggested meaning of scores (GDS-30): 0–4: normal, depending on age, education, complaints; 5–8: mild; 8–11: moderate; 12–15: severe; and thresholds for possible 'case' of depression ≥5 for GDS-15 and ≥2 for GDS-4.

Appendix 3

The patient health questionnaire (PHQ-9)

Name: ______________________________ Date: ____________________

Over the last 2 weeks, how often have you been bothered by any of the following problems? (Use '✓' to indicate your answer)

	Not at all	Several days	More than half the days	Nearly every day
1. Little interest or pleasure in doing things	0	1	2	3
2. Feeling down, depressed, or hopeless	0	1	2	3
3. Trouble falling or staying asleep, or sleeping too much	0	1	2	3
4. Feeling tired or having little energy	0	1	2	3
5. Poor appetite or overeating	0	1	2	3
6. Feeling bad about yourself—or that you are a failure or have let yourself or your family down	0	1	2	3
7. Trouble concentrating on things, such as reading the newspaper or watching television	0	1	2	3
8. Moving or speaking so slowly that other people could have noticed? Or the opposite—being so fidgety or restless that you have been moving around a lot more than usual	0	1	2	3
9. Thoughts that you would be better off dead or of hurting yourself in some way	0	1	2	3
Add columns	Total:			
10. If you checked off any problems, how difficult have these problems made it for you to do your work, take care of things at home, or get along with other people?	Not at all difficult ________ Somewhat difficult ________ Very difficult ________ Extremely difficult ________			

Appendix 2

The patient health questionnaire (PHQ-9)

Appendix 4

The World Health Organization well-being index

	Over the last 2 weeks	All of the time	Most of the time	More than half of the time	Less than half of the time	Some of the time	At no time
1	I have felt cheerful and in good spirits	❑ 5	❑ 4	❑ 3	❑ 2	❑ 1	❑ 0
2	I have felt calm and relaxed	❑ 5	❑ 4	❑ 3	❑ 2	❑ 1	❑ 0
3	I have felt active and vigorous	❑ 5	❑ 4	❑ 3	❑ 2	❑ 1	❑ 0
4	I woke up feeling fresh and rested	❑ 5	❑ 4	❑ 3	❑ 2	❑ 1	❑ 0
5	My daily life has been filled with things that interest me	❑ 5	❑ 4	❑ 3	❑ 2	❑ 1	❑ 0

Appendix 5

The Hamilton rating scale for depression

1 **DEPRESSED MOOD** *(sadness, hopeless, helpless, worthless)*

0 ❑ Absent
1 ❑ These feeling states indicated only on questioning
2 ❑ These feeling states spontaneously reported verbally
3 ❑ Communicates feeling states non-verbally, i.e. through facial expression, posture, voice, and tendency to weep
4 ❑ Patient reports virtually only these feeling states in his/her spontaneous verbal and non-verbal communication.

2 **FEELINGS OF GUILT**

0 ❑ Absent
1 ❑ Self-reproach, feels he/she has let people down
2 ❑ Ideas of guilt or rumination over past errors or sinful deeds
3 ❑ Present illness is a punishment. Delusions of guilt
4 ❑ Hears accusatory or denunciatory voices and/or experiences threatening visual hallucinations

3 **SUICIDE**

0 ❑ Absent
1 ❑ Feels life is not worth living
2 ❑ Wishes he/she were dead or any thoughts of possible death to self
3 ❑ Ideas or gestures of suicide
4 ❑ Attempts at suicide (any serious attempt rate 4)

4 **INSOMNIA: EARLY IN THE NIGHT**

0 ❑ No difficulty falling asleep
1 ❑ Complains of occasional difficulty falling asleep, i.e. more than half hour
2 ❑ Complains of nightly difficulty falling asleep

5 **INSOMNIA: MIDDLE OF THE NIGHT**

0 ❑ No difficulty
1 ❑ Patient complains of being restless and disturbed during the night
2 ❑ Waking during the night—any getting out of bed rates 2 (except for purposes of voiding)

6 **INSOMNIA: EARLY HOURS OF THE MORNING**

0 ❑ No difficulty
1 ❑ Waking in early hours of the morning but goes back to sleep
2 ❑ Unable to fall asleep again if he/she gets out of bed

7 **WORK AND ACTIVITIES**

0 ❑ No difficulty
1 ❑ Thoughts and feelings of incapacity, fatigue, or weakness related to activities, work, or hobbies
2 ❑ Loss of interest in activity, hobbies, or work—either directly reported by the patient or indirect in listlessness, indecision, and vacillation (feels he/she has to push self to work or activities)

3 ❑ Decrease in actual time spent in activities or decrease in productivity. Rate 3 if the patient does not spend at least 3 hours a day in activities (job or hobbies), excluding routine chores

4 ❑ Stopped working because of present illness. Rate 4 if patient engages in no activities, except routine chores, or if patient fails to perform routine chores unassisted

8 **RETARDATION** (slowness of thought and speech, impaired ability to concentrate, decreased motor activity)

0 ❑ Normal speech and thought

1 ❑ Slight retardation during the interview

2 ❑ Obvious retardation during the interview

3 ❑ Interview difficult

4 ❑ Complete stupor

9 **AGITATION**

0 ❑ None

1 ❑ Fidgetiness

2 ❑ Playing with hands, hair, etc.

3 ❑ Moving about, can't sit still

4 ❑ Hand wringing, nail biting, hair pulling, biting of lips

10 **ANXIETY PSYCHIC**

0 ❑ No difficulty

1 ❑ Subjective tension and irritability

2 ❑ Worrying about minor matters

3 ❑ Apprehensive attitude apparent in face or speech

4 ❑ Fears expressed without questioning

11 **ANXIETY SOMATIC (physiological concomitants of anxiety, such as:** gastro-intestinal—dry mouth, wind, indigestion, diarrhoea, cramps, belching; cardiovascular—palpitations; headaches; respiratory—hyperventilation, sighing; urinary frequency, sweating)

0 ❑ Absent

1 ❑ Mild

2 ❑ Moderate

3 ❑ Severe

4 ❑ Incapacitating

12 **SOMATIC SYMPTOMS GASTROINTESTINAL**

0 ❑ None

1 ❑ Loss of appetite but eating without staff encouragement. Heavy feelings in abdomen

2 ❑ Difficulty eating without staff urging. Requests or requires laxatives or medication for bowels or medication for gastrointestinal symptoms

13 **GENERAL SOMATIC SYMPTOMS**

0 ❑ None

1 ❑ Heaviness in limbs, back, or head. Backaches, headaches, muscle aches. Loss of energy and fatigability

2 ❑ Any clear-cut symptom rates 2

14 **GENITAL SYMPTOMS (symptoms such as loss of libido, menstrual disturbances)**

0 ❑ Absent.

1 ❑ Mild.

2 ❑ Severe.

15 **HYPOCHONDRIASIS**

0 ❑ Not present.

1 ❑ Self-absorption (bodily).

2 ❑ Preoccupation with health.

3 ❑ Frequent complaints, requests for help, etc.

4 ❑ Hypochondriacal delusions.

16 **LOSS OF WEIGHT (*RATE EITHER a OR b*)**

a) **According to the patient:**

0 ❑ No weight loss

1 ❑ Probable weight loss associated with present illness in week

2 ❑ Definite (according to patient) weight loss

b) **According to weekly measurements:**

0 ❑ Less than 1 lb in week.

1 ❑ Greater than 1 lb weight loss in week.

2 ❑ Greater than 2 lb weight loss in week

17 **INSIGHT**

0 ❑ Acknowledges being depressed and ill.

1 ❑ Acknowledges illness but attributes cause to bad food, climate, overwork, virus, need for rest, etc.

2 ❑ Denies being ill at all.

Total score: ❑❑

Appendix 6

Montgomery and Äsberg depression rating scale

1. Apparent sadness

Representing despondency, gloom, and despair (more than just ordinary transient low spirits), reflected in speech, facial expression, and posture. Rate by depth and inability to brighten up.

0 = No sadness ❑

2 = Looks dispirited but does brighten up without difficulty ❑

4 = Appears sad and unhappy most of the time ❑

6 = Looks miserable all the time. Extremely despondent ❑

2. Reported sadness

Representing reports of depressed mood, regardless of whether it is reflected in appearance or not.
Includes low spirits, despondency, or the feeling of being beyond help and without hope.

0 = Occasional sadness in keeping with the circumstances ❑

2 = Sad or low but brightens up without difficulty ❑

4 = Pervasive feelings of sadness or gloominess. The mood is still influenced by external circumstances ❑

6 = Continuous or unvarying sadness, misery, or despondency ❑

3. Inner tension

Representing feelings or ill-defined discomfort, edginess, inner turmoil, mental tension mounting to either panic, dread, or anguish. Rate according to intensity, frequency, duration, and the extent of reassurance called for.

0 = Placid. Only fleeting inner tension ❑

2 = Occasional feelings of edginess and ill-defined discomfort ❑

4 = Continuous feelings of inner tension or intermittent panic which the patient can only master with some difficulty ❑

6 = Unrelenting dread or anguish. Overwhelming panic ❑

4. Reduced sleep

Representing the experience of reduced duration or depth of sleep, compared to the subject's own normal pattern when well.

0 = Sleeps as usual ❑

2 = Slight difficulty dropping off to sleep or slightly reduced, light, or fitful sleep ❑

4 = Sleep reduced or broken by at least 2 hours ❑

6 = Less than 2 or 3 hours sleep ❑

5. Reduced appetite

Representing the feeling of a loss of appetite, compared with when well. Rate by loss of desire for food or the need to force oneself to eat.

0 = Normal or increased appetite ❑

2 = Slightly reduced appetite ❑

4 = No appetite. Food is tasteless ❑

6 = Needs persuasion to eat at all ❑

6. Concentration difficulties

Representing difficulties in collecting one's thoughts, mounting to an incapacitating lack of concentration. Rate according to intensity, frequency, and degree of incapacity produced.

0 = No difficulties in concentrating ❑

2 = Occasional difficulties in collecting one's thoughts ❑

4 = Difficulties in concentrating and sustaining thought which reduces ability to read or hold a conversation ❑

6 = Unable to read or converse without great difficulty ❑

7. Lassitude

Representing difficulty in getting started or slowness in initiating and performing everyday activities.

0 = Hardly any difficulty in getting started. No sluggishness ❑

2 = Difficulties in starting activities ❑

4 = Difficulties in starting simple routine activities, which are carried out with effort ❑

6 = Complete lassitude. Unable to do anything without help ❑

8. Inability to feel

Representing the subjective experience of reduced interest in the surroundings or activities that normally give pleasure. The ability to react with adequate emotion to circumstances or people is reduced.

0 = Normal interest in the surroundings and in other people ❑

2 = Reduced ability to enjoy usual interests ❑

4 = Loss of interest in the surroundings. Loss of feelings for friends and acquaintances ❑

6 = The experience of being emotionally paralysed, inability to feel anger, grief or pleasure, and a complete, or even painful, failure to feel for close relatives and friends ❑

9. Pessimistic thoughts

Representing thoughts of guilt, inferiority, self-reproach, sinfulness, remorse, and ruin.

0 = No pessimistic thoughts ❑

2 = Fluctuating ideas of failure, self-reproach, or self-depreciation ❑

4 = Persistent self-accusation or definite, but still rational, ideas of guilt or sin. Increasingly pessimistic about the future ❑

6 = Delusions of ruin, remorse, or irredeemable sin. Self-accusations, which are absurd and unshakable ❑

10. Suicidal thoughts

Representing the feeling that life is not worth living, that a natural death would be welcome, suicidal thoughts, and preparations for suicide. Suicide attempts should not in themselves influence the rating.

0 = Enjoys life or takes it as it comes ❑

2 = Weary of life. Only fleeting suicidal thoughts ❑

4 = Probably better off dead. Suicidal thoughts are common, and suicide is considered as a possible solution but without specific plans or intention ❑

6 = Explicit plans for suicide when there is an opportunity. Active preparations for suicide ❑

Appendix 7

Cornell scale for depression in dementia

Patient status:	❑ Nursing home resident	❑ Outpatient	❑ Inpatient
Informant used:	❑ Yes	❑ No	
Scores:	0 = absent	1 = mild or intermittent	2 = severe
	9999 = unable to evaluate		

Ratings should be based on symptoms and signs occurring during the week prior to interview.

If severe and intermittent, score as severe. No score should be given if symptoms result from physical disability or illness.

	INFORMANT				PATIENT				RATER'S OPINION			
A. MOOD-RELATED SIGNS												
1. ANXIETY Anxious expression, ruminations, worrying	0	1	2	9999	0	1	2	9999	0	1	2	9999
2. SADNESS Sad expression, sad voice, tearfulness	0	1	2	9999	0	1	2	9999	0	1	2	9999
3. LACK OF REACTIVITY TO PLEASANT EVENTS	0	1	2	9999	0	1	2	9999	0	1	2	9999
4. IRRITABILITY Easily annoyed, short-tempered	0	1	2	9999	0	1	2	9999	0	1	2	9999
B. BEHAVIOURAL DISTURBANCE												
5. AGITATION Restlessness, hand wringing, hair pulling	0	1	2	9999	0	1	2	9999	0	1	2	9999
6. RETARDATION Slow movements, slow speech, slow reactions	0	1	2	9999	0	1	2	9999	0	1	2	9999
7. MULTIPLE PHYSICAL COMPLAINTS (score 0 if GI symptoms only)	0	1	2	9999	0	1	2	9999	0	1	2	9999

8. LOSS OF INTEREST Less involved in usual activities (score only if change occurred acutely, i.e. in less than 1 month)	0	1	2	9999	0	1	2	9999	0	1	2	9999
C. PHYSICAL SIGNS												
9. APPETITE LOSS Eating less than usual	0	1	2	9999	0	1	2	9999	0	1	2	9999
10. WEIGHT LOSS (score 2 if greater than 5 lb in 1 month)	0	1	2	9999	0	1	2	9999	0	1	2	9999
11. LACK OF ENERGY Fatigues easily, unable to sustain activities (score only if change occurred acutely, i.e. in less than 1 month)	0	1	2	9999	0	1	2	9999	0	1	2	9999
D. CYCLIC FUNCTIONS												
12. DIURNAL VARIATION OF MOOD Symptoms worse in the morning	0	1	2	9999	0	1	2	9999	0	1	2	9999
13. DIFFICULTY FALLING ASLEEP Later than usual for this individual	0	1	2	9999	0	1	2	9999	0	1	2	9999
14. MULTIPLE AWAKENINGS DURING SLEEP	0	1	2	9999	0	1	2	9999	0	1	2	9999
15. EARLY MORNING AWAKENINGS Earlier than usual for this individual	0	1	2	9999	0	1	2	9999	0	1	2	9999
E. IDEATIONAL DISTURBANCE												
16. SUICIDE Feels life is not worth living, has suicidal wishes, or make suicide attempt	0	1	2	9999	0	1	2	9999	0	1	2	9999
17. SELF-DEPRECIATION Self-blame, poor self-esteem, feelings of failure	0	1	2	9999	0	1	2	9999	0	1	2	9999
18. PESSIMISM Anticipation of the worst	0	1	2	9999	0	1	2	9999	0	1	2	9999
19. MOOD-CONGRUENT DELUSIONS Delusions of poverty, illness, or loss	0	1	2	9999	0	1	2	9999	0	1	2	9999

Index

O

P

Q

R

S

T

U

V

W